Hygge

Danish Secrets to Happy Living

*(Scandinavian Ways of Living a Balanced Life
Filled With Coziness and Happiness)*

Michael Schultz

Published By **Elena Holly**

Michael Schultz

All Rights Reserved

*Hygge: Danish Secrets to Happy Living
(Scandinavian Ways of Living a Balanced Life
Filled With Coziness and Happiness)*

ISBN   978-1-7779502-8-6

No part of this guidebook shall be reproduced in any form without permission in writing from the publisher except in the case of brief quotations embodied in critical articles or reviews.

Legal & Disclaimer

The information contained in this book is not designed to replace or take the place of any form of medicine or professional medical advice. The information in this book has been provided for educational & entertainment purposes only.

The information contained in this book has been compiled from sources deemed reliable, and it is accurate to the best of the Author's knowledge; however, the Author cannot guarantee its accuracy and validity and cannot be held liable for any errors or omissions. Changes are periodically made to this book. You must consult your doctor or get professional medical advice before using any of the suggested remedies, techniques, or information in this book.

Table Of Contents

Chapter 1: The Five Dimensions............... 1

Chapter 2: The Ideal Living Space for
Effective Hygge Practice......................... 19

Chapter 3: Steamed Sugarloaf Cabbage . 37

Chapter 4: Healthy Hot Chocolate.......... 53

Chapter 5: Norwegian Porridge.............. 69

Chapter 6: Body Clothing and Covering.. 84

Chapter 7: Outdoor Practice 107

Chapter 8: The Workplace 117

Chapter 9: How to Make a Weekend
Routine 129

Chapter 10: Traditional Scandinavian
Dishes 133

Chapter 11: Scandinavian Design 141

Chapter 12: Scandinavian Lifestyle....... 154

Chapter 13: Scandinavian Folklore and
Mythology.. 166

Chapter 14: Scandinavian Festivals and Traditions... 172

Chapter 1: The Five Dimensions

Hygge is basically drama-loose devotedness time. It is cozying spherical, feeling loose and snug as one buries themselves in simplicity, warm temperature, and relaxation. But greater than that, it is being conscious that one's cushty time is sacred and treating it as such Because Danes see Hygge as this kind of important issue of suitable living, all of them art work together to make it occur. A lot of human beings count on it is approximately lighting candles, cooking up proper meals, and developing an thrilling surroundings. But that is terrific the ground function of Hygge. The reality is, Hygge is lots greater subterranean than that.

Below are five rules for powerful Hygge exercising? They will create a easy mental route to what the workout is all approximately, now not in fact on the ground however deep down in exercise.

Be real; come as you're

It is important to first be yourself and permit your defend down. You are not possibly to be criticized on Hygge territory, and doing so would now not be predicted of you each. When one strips themself of searching for to expose some component, they damage a ways from lies and sooner or later be part of in methods which may be plenty greater actual. Rivalry, conceitedness, and pretense are not bonding but as a substitute imperceptibly dividing.

Don't get stuck up inside the controversy.

Hygge is about a nicely-adjusted ebb and drift of debate in a snug fashion. The emphasis is on the moment and being in that 2d. There will usually be plenty of time in normal living to argue and deliberate, and experience the spectacle. However, Hygge is ready taking element within the meals and the employer and no longer getting caught up in topics that get rid of from that. As a quit end result, being cantankerous, closely pessimistic, judging, and quarreling are not allowed inside the hygge vicinity.

Embrace being a team member.

Everyone is aware what they will do to make a contribution without usually being probed. This makes the entire group waft better, and no one receives wedged doing all the paintings. When actually everybody works collectively in making, serving, pouring, and speaking, then Hygge is in complete shade. But all and sundry has to recognize that they're part of that team.

View Hygge as hotels from the out of doors.

Hygge time presents a provisional refuge from social mountaineering, networking, opposition, and materialism. It is an area wherein every person can loosen up and open their hearts with out arbitrating, regardless of the contemporary-day happenings of their lifestyles. This is particular because it we could families and friends usually be able to connect on this vicinity without the horrors of judgment. This region is blessed for specific or lousy, and snags may be disregarded of doorways.

Have in mind that it's time-constrained

Making hygge may be perplexing for a non-Dane. No one takes center degree, no person brags or complains, no unfold of negativity, and every person tries to be gift without quarreling. This can be difficult to do for quite some households. But the remuneration is massive. It feels high-quality to percentage the ones drama-unfastened moments with the ones one cares approximately. It is a remarkable deal less complicated to try to experience that second if one knows that it's far virtually going on for that particular dinner, lunch, or quick time. The fact is that one's troubles is probably watching for them outside Hygge's door when they depart. But they may be capable of wait outside for a touch at the same time as for some issue larger.

HYGGE FOR THE SENSES

The scent of hygge.

Anything sweet and uplifting to you is the perfume of hygge. It is probably the iconic odor of glowing homemade baked devices, or it could be an aroma that is extra uncommon than excellent you could apprehend. Furthermore, the Hygge heady scent is probably the scent of 1's domestic, maybe their bed room, as it triggers their senses of safety and ease.

The taste of hygge.

The flavor of hygge is some thing candy and comforting. This can range from what one eats that triggers happy memories and emotions to what one beverages that motive relaxation and heat. The Hygge smell also binds one to the atmospheres of freedom and tranquillity.

The sounds of hygge.

The sounds of hygge essentially hyperlink with the nonattendance of sound, some factor like a paradox of a few type. With the absence of sound, it is straightforward to better concentrate the small comforting sounds, together with the sizzling of timber in the hearth, raindrops on the roof, the sound of the wind outside on a blustery day, or possibly the chirrup of the crickets on summer season dusks. Any sound that one friends with a stable and comforting setting can be hygge.

The revel in of hygge.

The feeling of hygge can be corporeal, or it may be figurative. Handmade antique subjects will typically be picked over artificial subjects at the same time as denoting a few element that is hyggelig. The sense of some issue weathered, herbal, or rustic will commonly be associated with Hygge. Another chief a part of feeling hygge is being cushty and secure in an adverse environment. Now, this may appear a hint immoderate. However, this is in reference to the kind of consolation one memories whilst the wintry climate winds are whistling outdoor while one is relaxed and warmth inside; or whilst one is curled up of their bed at night time time time below the covers, and it's far barely frosty outside of these covers. All of these emotions talk with the feeling of hygge.

Seeing hygge.

It might be hard to try and envision some thing this is particularly primarily based completely at the manner one feels. The awesome aspect about the artwork of Hygge is that feasible envision it further to enjoy it. The Danes take remarkable satisfaction in their lighting fixtures, which performs a primary component in envisioning hygge. Dimmed and clean lighting fixtures is top in case you need to have a 2d of hygge, see hygge, in addition to experience it. Also, Hygge values slow tempo residing. It is ready taking it sluggish. Watch matters circulate genuinely slowly, just like the falling snow or the tongues of flames slowly licking up the last coals in a fireplace. A visualization of hygge is pastoral, dim, and gradual.

INSTANT HYGGE

DEEP CONNECTIONS THROUGH COZINESS

When someone makes a selection to embark at the excellent adventure of working in the direction of Hygge, developing coziness in a single's existence, they begin to experience a depth of that means that they'd hitherto won't be professional without it in advance than. This will in addition go past to emotions of happiness and contentment as soon as the path of 1's life starts offevolved offevolved to alternate for the higher, and with one's project and the people in their existence, one will become enabled to move ahead on their path. As one will become familiar with the added remunerations coziness offers, one additionally appreciates that obtaining relaxed is a terrific way to further find out the real because of this of lifestyles.

LET'S GET COZY FOR COMFORT.

A suitable way to provide an reason for coziness is that it's miles all about being comfortable. Once one is snug, one feels a warmness feeling deep interior, and everything starts offevolved to sense right inside their global. There are some of procedures to recognize the consolation of coziness after being at ease with one's surroundings, with themself, and with others.

When someone is cushty in their surroundings, they sense regular and sheltered. When they may be confronted with being in a brand new placing, they every now and then go through a time of adjustment wherein they're not one hundred% relaxed. This frequently comes approximately after they bypass to a contemporary city, begin a cutting-edge hobby, or visit a new domestic. If one is resuming a new activity, it is probably of high-quality assist for them to check the modern-day facility and the people they might be strolling with there earlier than their first day. This must useful resource them in attending to experience more cushty. Once they get into their new feature, they may lightly switch to feeling extra comfortable as each day passes. So, setting strive into attempting to speak to one's new colleagues and bearing on with them on a deeper diploma will help the person thru the transition. In addition, being with out issues on hand and open will aid co-employees in mastering one better, and, hopefully, they will talk in self notion to them as well.

SELF-COMFORT

Being snug in a single's pores and pores and skin includes that the individual is present and living within the now of their life; they will be whole of positivity and simply like themself. Little subjects do not get into one's head, thereby distorting their stability and emotions, and one feels a feel of tranquility no matter what they may be worried in. It is a fashionable feeling that everything is as lots as scratch in a single's global. When a person like themself, they do not worry and are self-confident approximately their options. Consequently, other mother and father will feel interested by them as they emanate a sturdy experience of positivity. Typically, they will be assured and cross after their dreams in vicinity of looking for his or her desires to miraculously seem earlier than them. Despite the fact that such a person is a pass-getter, they by no means appear to be overly strained out via occasions that can get up. They are an encouragement to themselves and others. Being cushty with one's self consists of being cushty and content material in a single's devoutness, knowing the course one has determined on to walk on, and knowledge that there are schoolings in each revel in.

Coziness moreover implies being cushty with one-of-a-type humans. If one is overly shy, there are a number of strategies to enjoy more snug interacting with others.

1.   First, it is essential to hold eye contact with people whilst talking with them. This act establishes a reference to them and makes them appear self-confident of their interactions, irrespective of the reality that

they are feeling uncomfortable on the internal. The greater one runs thru this, the an lousy lot much less uncomfortable one starts offevolved to feel. However, one has to attempt now not to stare someone down as then one might cause them to uncomfortable.

2.   Second, pay particular interest to the frame language of numerous human beings and the manner they act in reaction to at the least one's moves or phrases. This will assist one decide their subsequent line of motion due to that.

Bringing a experience of coziness to at least one's self, paintings, and different people will boom their positivity and happy moments in lifestyles. From time to time, this could take a piece art work, however it is genuinely really worth the attempt. If one makes it a practice to be useful in place of estranging themselves from brilliant people whom they percentage similar paths with, it is able to add deeper due to this and a sense of coziness to at least one's life, developing absolutely satisfied research for themselves and others; ultimately, no individual is going via lifestyles on my own as every body have own family, pals, and instructors. We are related to loads of people in the course of our lifetime. Some of those humans might be worried with us for our whole existence, at the same time as others come and circulate after a brief even as.

LIGHTS AND CANDLES

It is a truth that no steering for Hygge is taken into consideration enough with out candles. A poll as soon as confirmed that after Danes have been asked what they associate most with Hygge, an awe-inspiring 80 five percent stated candles.

Lyseslukker is a Danish word used to provide an explanation for one that locations out the candles, and that is no twist of destiny. There isn't always any quicker way to motive Hygge than to slight some candles or lavenders, or dwelling lights (as fondly noted in Danish). The Danes usually love undertakings with candles; it is not simply candles in their living rooms; it's far everywhere, from their school rooms to their boardrooms. It breeds a form of emotional delight, an emotional coziness.

Statistically, every Dane burns spherical thirteen kilos of candle wax every one year; and Denmark burns greater candles in keeping with head than any region inside the entire of Europe (this is in line with the European Candle Association). This candle consumption is a European document. In reality, Denmark burns nearly instances as masses candle wax as 2d-located Austria, with a piece below seven pounds in keeping with 365 days. Nevertheless, scented candles are not a massive difficulty (that is true, due to the fact the oldest producer of candles in Denmark might no longer even include scented candles of their product variety). Scented candles are labeled as non-herbal, and Danes pick out natural and natural products. In reality, even as it comes to shopping for herbal merchandise, Danes rank at the top of the listing in all of Europe.

LAMPS

Even despite the fact that Danes are infatuated with lighting in popular, for them, lighting fixtures is not really approximately candles. Danes handpick lamps with judgment and location them tactically to fashion calming swimming swimming pools of moderate. It is an art work shape, a talent, and a exchange. Some of the most gorgeously designed lamps inside the international have their roots and origins inside the golden age of Danish designs (a few pinnacle examples encompass the lamps of Poul Henningsen, Arne Jacobsen, and Verner Panton).

As a intellectual check, one ought to continually pass for lights that emit lower temperatures, as this is considered to be greater Hygge. A virtual digicam flash emits about 5,500 Kelvin of power; a fluorescent tube emits spherical five,000K; an incandescent lamp emits 3,000K, at the identical time as sunsets, timber, and candle flames are about 1,800K. It is critical to discover the candy spot for one's hygge enjoy.

The Danish have some of lamps that could be considered iconic.

The PH lamp: After about ten years of experimenting with diverse lamps and lights in his loft, Henningsen unveiled the primary PH lamp in 1925. This lamp emitted a softer and mellower slight by way of using the usage of a chain of encrusted shades to scatter the mild yet masks the moderate bulb. Furthermore, to convey the merciless white mild toward the crimson quit of the continuum, PH gave the inner flank of 1 element of the color a red color. His crucial success grow to be PH5, which had metal sun shades and have become launched in 1958; however, PH lamps have now been produced in over 1000 severa designs. A lot of these are not in production anymore, and the rarest lamps can pass for delivered than $25,000 at public sale.

Le Klint lamps

The engineer, architect, and painter, P.V. Jensen Klint, designed the first actual mild shade, and afterward, his sons, Kaare and Tage Klint sustained his works, making Le Klint a organization well-known for its sought-after classics in addition to its constantly renewing and emergent choice.

Le Klint's hand-folded slight sunglasses and suspended lamps, made in Le Klint's commercial enterprise unit in Odense, Denmark, are sought-after cutting-edge classics that glide well with some of awesome interiors. The dexterously hand-customary, awesome slight sun shades are concurrently ageless and in style, with a number of the designs, similar to the only 0 one designed through Kaare Klint, dating again to the 1940s.

Photography

Photographers might be honestly as infatuated with lights as the Danes. Photography is a sort of painting, except it's miles with mild. Indulging in snap shots will growth one's draw near of slight and their capability to appearance and respect it. Photographers are given to take tens of plenty of pix time and again. Some of them choose the golden hour, which takes area about one hour earlier than dawn and an hour earlier than sunset. When the sun is low within the sky, the sunlight journeys through a extra intensity of surroundings. During those times, it creates a heat, tender, diffused slight. It is occasionally furthermore known as the magic hour. One need to intention for this mild if they'll be going for hyggelig lighting fixtures indoors.

Chapter 2: The Ideal Living Space for Effective Hygge Practice

For certainly all and sundry, dwelling a comfortable life can be a completely non-public state of affairs, differing from man or woman to individual This manner that what feels relaxed to as a minimum one won't sense relaxed to another. One way to discover one's personal options a deep spiritual stroll can also ought to be launched into. This will necessarily loose up the wanted expertise approximately one's spiritual self and the way coziness can help them benefit each their non-public and non secular ends.

HYGGE CEREMONIALS TO INTRODUCE INTO ONE'S LIFE

Lighting

Begin with dimming the lighting fixtures and digging out the candles. It is first-class to go for herbal beeswax candles over scented ones. Suitable lighting fixtures is an essential part of Hygge. Soft, herbal glows propose a warmer and additional calming environment.

If you do no longer have candles, there may be no want to be discouraged. One can without a doubt turn off the extraordinary and illuminating lights and skip for incredible-toned lamps or fairy lighting fixtures to intensify warm temperature and coziness.

Hygge with buddies and own family

The remarkable of Hygge is gotten at the same time as it is shared with a near organisation of people. Lessons drawn have indicated that spending precious time with cherished ones makes us the happiest. Meet with friends and family over a heat cup of chocolate, sit down throughout the desk and serve a heat meal, play board video video games collectively, or chat and giggle until the wee hours of the morning. Hilarity, communicate, and warmth of friendship are all part of Hygge.

Cozy styles of Stuff

You can style hygge in your own home with the resource of breaking out the blankets and pillows, laying significance on subjects herbal and clean, if possible, made from herbal substances which incorporates wool. You can fashion a cushty area of interest with clean hassocks and blankets in which you could snuggle up with a great e-book. Hygge is all about feeling at home and fashioning an area with pieces that make you satisfied.

Be Comfortable

Achieving consolation is simple; in reality think about knit sweaters, woolly socks, and heat leggings. Adopting herbal fibers is a fantastic approach to feeling warmth and comfortable at a few degree in the pointy wintry weather. One can dig up their preferred warmth and relaxed clothes and get prepared to hygge.

Prioritize healthy eating and drinking.

One essential a part of Hygge is pandering to the good stuff in lifestyles. For masses of humans, this includes first rate, comforting, and hearty food. It is essential to preserve food smooth and spend time with cherished ones via getting prepared meals together. Hygge is ready nourishing one's flavor buds and allowing one's self to revel in things that bring about happiness. Loaves, pastries, and cookies are in truth hygge. Also, serve up the ones heat beverages inclusive of mugs of tea, wealthy warm cocoa, and espresso. These are all correct for warming the soul.

Unplug

Living inside the 2d and embracing life is the bedrock of Hygge. So, you may acquire those thru turning off cell telephones and television and as an opportunity sharing a verbal exchange with close to pals or family, choosing up an excellent e-book, being attentive to or developing appropriate track, painting a picture of nature or a few shape of artwork, or gambling a board exercise. One of the very quality matters to get lost in is the virtual global; this will motive one neglecting themselves and others. One want to spend time with themselves or the human beings one cherishes. One can choose to quickly eliminate shows as they function full-size distractions from being gift and within the second.

Link with Nature

As an entire lot as Hygge is ready fashioning a heat and inviting indoor place, it's far a regarded reality that Danes enjoy all seasons and getting out often. Hygge is set equilibrium and generating a healthy existence. This is why exposure to nature is critical. Spending time outdoor is commonly quite smooth; whilst immersed in nature, one is probably to be extra present and cushty.

Introduce nature for your interior.

One detail nature may not lack is happiness. This is why bringing the outside interior is a extraordinary manner to enjoy associated with the outdoor on the identical time as final snuggly internal. Bunches of glowing blooms, fir cones, willowy branches, and masses of wooden are all cues of our lovely global outside. Feeling allied to nature, even signs and symptoms and signs of it indoors, aids in bringing a experience of peace and luxury.

Create a Fire

While the temperature falls outdoor, a roaring hearth is one of the few matters which can evoke the sensation of coziness. This can draw dad and mom in like an abstraction at the equal time as embossing a revel in of calm and peace. A right Hygge fire ought to use actual wooden.

Hang on

Hygge is relishing and taking detail in the instant. So, preserve near on after food, revel in conversations, and sluggish the pace of life. Pour your self a cup of heat cocoa, light some lighting, cuddle up with someone specific, and take it all in carefully. Aim to gain this enlightenment with coziness, companionship, and delight. You can add a bit Hygge on your existence and include the season's beauties.

HYGGE DÉCOR: GUIDELINES TO HYGGE YOUR HOME

The ideology behind the Hygge workout is to efficaciously create a secure residing area for oneself, their friends, and own family. With the season of own family gatherings doping up now after which, there's no impeccable time to Hygge one's domestic. When beautifying and redecorating your living vicinity, one want to now not lose sight of simplicity; this is crucial if one have to submerge their self on this lighthearted and comfortable way of life. Below is a listing of a few techniques you will be capable of create Hygge of their domestic, some few activities and some others to keep away from as a amazing deal as feasible.

Natural shade schemes are remarkable. Stay with them.

An overwhelming shade scheme can be bad to Hygge. This is why one is usually recommended to hold them easy. Everything added to as a minimum one's Hygge domestic want to add to an atmosphere of accord and peace. Going with a unbiased coloration palette is vital whilst growing a space that induces relaxation. Using pastel colours such as light greys, browns, and creams will fashion a peaceful region for one and their site visitors to enjoy.

Create a comfortable environment.

Remember that the primary consciousness of Hygge ornament is constantly coziness. One way to do that is by way of adorning with feathery pillows and easy duvets. Snuggle up on the couch with blankets, cushions, and pillows to create a snug vicinity to unwind. One can also do that through fashioning cushty nooks like a window bench or a loveseat. These have to feature suitable spots to loosen up with an remarkable ebook and a cup of heat cocoa.

Employ the usage of candles to beautify.

Candles are strongly associated with romance, rest, prayers, and so forth. Hygge additionally has deep connections to lights and candles. This enables with evoking an surroundings of calm, tranquility, and rest. The indulgent and mild glow of a candle can not be simulated via the use of the usage of something else and need to be used for the duration of one's home to style a warm temperature vivacity.

Employ twinkly lights to moderate up the place.

Twinkly lighting are considered idyllic with regards to hygge ornamentation. Not satisfactory are they jolly and celebratory, but they look extraordinary anywhere within the region. They may be utilized in a unmarried's bed room, residing room, or possibly an outdoor courtyard. These lights, like candles, emit a softer slight and complement an fun touch to at least one's home layout without being too prodigious.

Textures are critical. Add them in.

When one ponders cushty Hygge décor, the feel won't efficiently come to mind. But bringing texture to at least one's residing area is a fantastic manner to decorate hobby in an in any other case minimalist scheme. This may be finished by way of way of integrating warmness, herbal factors which includes timber and wool into one's ornament. Flowers may be incorporated for variability and a modest splash of color.

Redesign your relaxation room to be spa-fashion.

As an possibility to really the use of one's relaxation room for short showers inside the morning, one's toilet can be an area for relaxation and rejuvenation. To style an a laugh and non violent bathroom, one has to make certain that they've lots of hidden garage areas to avoid any unsolicited clutter. For greater pleasure, you will put money into candles and comfortable robes for a laid-lower lower back and tranquil design.

What to do:

Arrange ornaments with awesome styles of candles for the duration of your area to create a heat and relaxed surroundings.

Stick to soothing pastels and neutrals like greys, creams, and browns.

Decorate with blankets, fluffy pillows, and cushty sofas and seats.

Utilize your hearth as a huge issue for accumulating with friends and own family.

Adorn your place with quite lighting that brighten and add warm temperature.

Create a chilled surroundings for your rest room with a spa-style bathtub.

Incorporate natural substances along with wood, wool, and diverse styles of plant life.

What not to do:

Avoid the use of candles with overpowering fragrances.

Avoid combining excessively exquisite and stale-setting shades for your decorations.

Refrain from the usage of cutting-edge-fashion furniture and limiting seating options.

Don't regard your fireplace absolutely as an embellishment; preserve in mind it a focus for accumulating.

Avoid using large and super lamps that produce a harsh glow.

Don't reflect onconsideration on your bathroom most effective as a convenience; create a area for rest.

Avoid which include vibrant designs and textures that disrupt the general aesthetics.

FOODS, DRINKS, AND THE 'HOW'S.'

Food and liquids for Hygge

Food and drinks are a essential a part of the Hygge workout. This is due to the truth getting and feeling as comfy and satisfied as feasible includes a devotion to ingesting and ingesting, which offers to one's happiness. Hygge recipes are not sincerely any antique consolation substances. Even despite the fact that they may be certainly licentious and warming, they need to be pretty smooth to make, exciting, mild, nutritious, and healthy.

There are a gaggle of recipes that you in all likelihood can probe for experiencing a Hygge in food and drink. These recipes trigger the Hygge enjoy in spell binding and although judiciously wholesome methods. It is a truth that actual pleasures are frequently placed inside the commonplaces of our normal dwelling. Below are some authentically scrumptious thoughts to deliver Hygge closer to one's residing region.

HYGGE FOODS

Poached Salmon with Cucumber Pickle and Dill Crème Fraiche.

Ingredients (for 6 servings)

For the salmon:

600g aspect of salmon

1 sliced onion

1 sliced lemon

four tbsp caster sugar

½ Tbsp salt

2 handfuls of dill

50ml white wine (for the cucumber pickle)

4 tbsp cider vinegar

1 small shallot

1 cucumber

For the dill crème fraîche:

A handful of dill

200g crème fraîche

½ Piece of lemon juice

Baby potatoes

How to prepare

Begin via preheating the oven to one hundred
and eighty°C/350°F/Gas Mark.

Place the onion and lemon slices in a massive roasting tray and feature sprigs of dill over the top.

Place the salmon over and season with sea salt, milled black pepper, and a very last trickle of dill.

Pour water and wine everywhere inside the sides of the salmon and cowl the roasting tray with tin foil.

Place the roasting tray within the oven for 15 minutes or until certainly cooked via.

Mix the sugar and vinegar in a bowl for the cucumber pickle until the sugar has honestly melted.

Mix within the salt and shallot, then upload the thin slices of cucumber.

Cover this aggregate and refrigerate for as a minimum 2 hours or in a single day.

Mix the dill, Creme Fraiche, a snap of black pepper, and lemon juice.

Finally, dish the cooked salmon with the cucumber pickle, Creme Fraiche, and a few freshly cooked little one potatoes on a plate.

Toasted Coconut Breakfast Porridge

Ingredients (for five servings)

14 oz. Of coconut milk

half of of of cup of Quinoa

A pinch of salt

1.50 cups of rolled oats

1 cup of juice or water (bai5 antioxidant infusions Congo pear

Half a cup of unsweetened coconut flakes

Cinnamon (to taste)

Apple slices, peanut butter, or honey (for topping options)

How to prepare

Using a small saucepan, convey the coconut milk to a boil.

Add the quinoa and salt. Cook for 15 minutes till the quinoa is cooked.

Add the Bai5, oats, cinnamon, and salt. These can put together dinner for only a few extra mins to melt the oats.

Using medium-immoderate warm temperature, upload the coconut flakes to a small nonstick skillet. Shake inside the pan till lightly toasted. This can also be finished within the oven; however, the stovetop is faster.

Serve the porridge with toasted coconut or each other topping making a decision on.

Use 1/2 of a cup of the Bai5 for a thicker consistency.

Add a whole cup for a much lighter and softer porridge. One can start through which include half cup first and then upload greater because the combination soaks up greater wetness.

Note: One can pick out to feature in different forms of seeds or grains. For instance, it is simple to use 1 cup of quinoa and half of freekeh. However, one has to discern out the amount of time and quantity of water the ones grains require to put together dinner dinner nicely.

Chapter 3: Steamed Sugarloaf Cabbage

Ingredients (for 4 servings)

Steamed sugarloaf cabbage:

250g of unsalted butter

1 piece of sugarloaf cabbage, tough outer layers removed and rinsed

Sea salt to flavor

2 tablespoons of freshly grated horseradish

Dill sprigs to serve

Salted lemon rind:

1 herbal lemon

1 tablespoon of sea salt

How to put together

For the salted lemon rind:

Peel the lemon first, and then located the rind and salt in a zipper-top bag.

Toss well, after which stand for at the least 2 hours or in a single day.

Rinse off the salt, pat dry the rind, and finely chop.

Melt 150g butter in a small pan over low heat, making sure it does not boil.

Take out the clean butter from the pinnacle and region it in a smooth pan. Remove the milk solids resting at the bottom of the pan as well.

Melt the butter in a medium-sized saucepan over medium-high warm temperature till it acquires a nutty mild brown shade, then take it off the heat.

As you prepare the cabbage, go away it apart to relax.

For the sugarloaf cabbage:

Cut the cabbage into 4-6 wedges.

To soften the butter, set a good sized frying pan over medium warm temperature. Shake the pan until the butter melts, then add 100g of butter, salt, and some water splashes.

Add the cabbage wedges next. Then cowl the pan with a lid or a bit of foil and steam the cabbage wedges for approximately 2 mins.

Open the pan and flip the cabbage to the opposite issue. Cover and steam for a few other 2 mins or until the cabbage is clean. The cooking time is based upon on the scale of the cabbage.

Place the warm cabbage on a big serving dish. Mix the chopped salted lemon rind and horseradish into the brilliant and cushty burned butter and season with sea salt.

Serve the burned butter over the cabbage, ensuring it runs down all of the layers.

Scatter with dill sprigs and a hint greater grated horseradish if desired, and then serve right now.

Note: Sugarloaf cabbage has a totally specific narrowed-fashioned head and is favored for its gentle, clean and sweet leaves. If one can not get this, a small Savoy cabbage may be used as an opportunity.

Slow Cooked Scottish Beef Stew

Ingredients (for 4 servings)

For beef stew:

2 tablespoons of butter or coconut oil

1 massive chopped onion

700g of red meat shin (cubed and further fats removed)

3 big carrots chopped into chunks

1 small turnip chopped into pieces

1 garlic clove

1 cup of flour

4 cups of water

Red currant jelly

Red wine

Salt & pepper

Optional: mashed potatoes, kale, broccoli, and many others.

To serve:

Fresh thyme sprigs

Fresh bread

How to put together

Begin thru preheating the oven to 160c/325f

Heat the oil in a big pan. Fry the pork for 7-8 minutes until golden brown after being dusted with flour.

Add the onions and garlic; put together dinner dinner for a in addition five mins

Add the redcurrant jelly, then pour in the pink wine and simmer for five minutes

Add the salt, pepper, kale, broccoli, and carrots.

Bring to a gradual boil, then cowl; put together dinner within the oven for 3-4 hours.

Ensure that it is stirred several instances all through cooking; a few exclusive desire is to exchange it to a gradual cooker and cook it on high or low for 5-6 or 7-eight hours, respectively.

Garnish with freshly reduce bread and a hint sparkling thyme.

Vegan cut up pea soup with dill and crispy onions

Ingredients (for four servings)

2 tsps. Of olive oil

2 medium-sized yellow onions, chopped

2 medium-sized celery stalks, diced

2 medium-sized carrots, diced

¼ medium sized celery root, diced

6 cups vegetable inventory

2 cups of dried inexperienced cut up peas

1 sprig of sparkling thyme

four tsps. Of chopped glowing dill

2 medium-sized yellow onions sliced salt and pepper

How to prepare

Begin thru heating the olive oil in a soup pot over medium-immoderate warm temperature.

Add the chopped onions and sauté; heat for approximately 15 mins or till golden.

Add the onions, celery stalks, carrots, celery root, vegetable inventory, dried inexperienced split peas, sparkling thyme, and 1/2 of of the dill. Bring to a boil.

After turning down the warm temperature, cowl the pot, and simmer it for forty five minutes until the peas are mild and the soup is aromatic.

Meanwhile, sauté the sliced onions in a skillet over medium-immoderate warmth until darkened and crispy.

Remove from skillet and set apart for topping.

Season soup with salt and pepper.

Serve crowned with crispy onions and smooth dill.

Notes: If celery root is unavailable, you may use rutabaga, turnip, or parsnip.

Vegan Pumpkin Cinnamon Rolls

Ingredients (for four servings)

DOUGH:

1 cup of unsweetened almond milk

2 tablespoons of vegan butter

1 packet (~2 1/4 teaspoons) of immediately yeast

1 tablespoon of herbal cane sugar

1/4 teaspoon of sea salt

half of teaspoon of cinnamon

1 teaspoon of pumpkin pie spice

1/three cup of pumpkin puree

2 three/4–3 1/4 cups of Unbleached All-Purpose Flour

FILLING:

2 half of of tablespoons of vegan butter

half cup of pumpkin butter

1/3 cup of organic cane sugar

1 tablespoon of cinnamon

1/2 of teaspoon of pumpkin pie spice

half of of cup of uncooked pecans, chopped (optionally to be had)

TOPPING:

2 tablespoons of vegan butter

1 tablespoon of pumpkin butter (optionally available)

1 tablespoon of herbal cane sugar

1/4 cup of raw pecans

How to put together

For the dough:

Begin through way of heating the almond milk and vegan butter in a pan over medium warmth; this have to be finished in 30-second increments till warmth and melted. It should now not boil.

Remove from stovetop and allow cool to a hundred and ten°F (40 3°C); this is about the temperature of bathtub water. This is critical in order now not to kill the yeast.

If warmed at the stovetop, transfer the aggregate to a huge mixing bowl.

Dust on yeast, sugar, and salt and allow to affect for ten minutes.

Add the cinnamon and pumpkin pie spice, after which combination. Let it set for a couple of minutes.

Whip the pumpkin purée on the equal time as adding it to the combination.

Next, whisk inside the flour (half a cup at a time). Consistently stir at the same time as you add the flour.

Transfer the dough to a gently floured ground and knead until it workplace work a unfastened ball, which includes flour as wanted.

Rinse and coat the mixture bowl with oil. Put the dough ball lower returned inside the bowl and roll it round to gently coat it. Wrap the dough in plastic wrap and vicinity it in a warmth location for 40-five mins till it has doubled in period.

Roll the dough into a thin rectangle on a gently floured ground.

For the Filling:

Brush with heated vegan butter and pumpkin butter, and then upload sugar, cinnamon, pumpkin pie spice, and pecans.

Beginning at one surrender, tightly roll up the dough and position the seam side down.

Then, with a jagged knife, reduce the dough into 1.Five–2-inch sections and role it in a well-lubricated pan.

For the Garnishings:

Brush with vegan butter combined with pumpkin butter; dust with cane sugar and pecans, and cowl with plastic wrap.

Set on pinnacle of the oven and permit it upward push once more whilst preheating the oven to 350°F (176°C).

Once the oven is warm, bake the rolls on a middle rack for 30-forty minutes or till golden brown (crusty on top).

Let cool for at least 10 mins earlier than serving.

Cinnamon rolls should be saved included at room temperature for a few days. One can freeze dough reduce it into cinnamon rolls, and vicinity it in a pan.

Cover nicely and freeze in a pan, then allow it defrost for as a minimum 6 hours in advance than baking.

Cover and set on pinnacle of the preheated oven to rise; then bake.

Notes:

Pumpkin butter can both be provided at the shop or made at home. If one does purchase, make sure that they will be vegan-pleasant.

For a simple dairy-loose glaze-

Melt 1 tsp. Vegan butter and whisk in half of of cup powdered or finely floor sugar.

Thin with 1 tsp of dairy-unfastened milk at a time till thick but pourable.

Add 1 tablespoon of pumpkin butter and 1/4 tsp. Of pumpkin pie spice for extra pumpkin taste.

(Kanelbullar) Swedish Cinnamon Buns Recipe

Ingredients (for 4 servings)

1.2 cups of almond milk or complete milk

1 package deal (2 1/four tsp.) of lively dry yeast

1/2 cup of unrefined granulated sugar

1 huge egg; 1 egg yolk

four tsps. Of vanilla bean, paste or extract

3 tsps. Of ground cardamom

2 tsps. Of kosher salt

3 ½ - four cups of unbleached flour

1 stick (8 tsp.) of unsalted butter at room temperature

half of of cup of mild brown sugar

4 tsps. Of floor cinnamon

Toasted sliced almonds or pearl sugar for garnish

How to put together

Making the Foam:

Begin with the resource of heating the milk to one hundred ten° to one hundred fifteen°F and then add the yeast and a pinch of granulated sugar to the stand mixer bowl. Set apart for about five to 10 mins or until foamy.

Add half cup of granulated sugar, the egg and egg yolk, 2 teaspoons of vanilla, 2 teaspoons of cardamom, and a couple of teaspoons of salt, and then whisk until well combined.

For the Dough:

Slowly add 3 half cups of all-motive flour to the stand mixer prepared with a dough hook and knead till a slight silky dough paperwork. The dough should be sticky, silky, and slack enough to fall on itself when set down slightly.

If the dough sticks to the hands after 3 half of cups, add the remaining 1 cup flour in periods of tablespoons till the preferred consistency is gotten.

Mix in 4 tablespoons of butter, some quantities at a time, till well mixed.

Shape the dough proper right into a ball, pushing the ends below so the top ground is suave.

Allowing the Dough to Rise:

Lightly spray a smooth bowl with nonstick spray and roll the dough ball in oil.

Cover with plastic wrap or a moist kitchen towel, and set in a heat location for about forty five minutes to at least one hour at room temperature or in a single day within the fridge; permit to upward push till doubled.

When geared up to form the cinnamon rolls, make the filling by the use of manner of mixing the final 4 tsp. Of butter, 1/four cup of moderate brown sugar, three tsp. Of ground cinnamon, half of of tsp. Of ground cardamom, a pinch of salt, and half of tsp. Of vanilla bean paste. Stir till thoroughly combined.

Chapter 4: Healthy Hot Chocolate

Ingredients (for four servings)

Hot chocolate:

2 half of of cups of unsweetened almond milk

2 teaspoons of cacao powder

1 teaspoon of Maca powder

2 teaspoons of maple syrup

half teaspoon of coconut oil

Pinch of cinnamon

Tiny pinch of sea salt

Optional toppings:

Coconut whip

Shaved dark chocolate

How to prepare

Begin with the useful aid of mixing the almond milk, cacao powder, maca, maple syrup, coconut oil, cinnamon, and salt in a blender. This can also be whisked collectively by means of the use of hand.

Transfer to a small pan and warmth over medium warmth. Taste and awesome-music the surprise if favored. If too thick, upload a bit greater almond milk.

Serve with coconut whip and shaved dark chocolate.

Notes:

Homemade Coconut Whip: solids from 1 can of entire-fat coconut milk, refrigerated in a unmarried day; ⅓cup of powdered sugar, and some drops of vanilla extract.

Grilled red meat stomach with parsley sauce

Ingredients (for 4 servings)

Pork belly:

800g of boneless red meat stomach, sliced into 1cm huge quantities

1 tablespoon of olive oil

1kg of Kipfler potatoes

2 tablespoons of salt

Sea salt flakes for seasoning

Parsley sauce:

50g of butter

35g (¼ cup) of plain flour

500ml (2 cups) of milk

½ teaspoon of salt

½ cup of finely shredded curly or flat-leaf parsley, plus more for serving

Freshly ground black pepper

1.   How to put together

Begin via manner of preheating the oven to 200°C.

Place pork on a rack and set it inside the roasting tray.

Brush the beef with oil and season with sea salt flakes.

Ensure it chefs for forty minutes or until the beef is golden and crisp, flipping it midway via.

Take it out of the oven and loosely cover it with foil. Set aside for five minutes to rest.

While the beef is resting, located the potatoes in a large pan with smooth cold water. Season with salt and permit it to boil. Ensure the potatoes are cooked for fifteen minutes or until they're easy whilst poked with a skewer. Drain the water and allow it to dry in the pan with the lid off.

Making the parsley sauce:

The first step will be to soften butter in a saucepan on medium warmth. Add in flour and allow it put together dinner dinner for a minute. Next, slowly stir within the bloodless milk, then permit it to simmer. Stir constantly till the sauce has thickened in your selected consistency.

Season with salt and pepper, then mix through the parsley.

Serve the potatoes and pork with the parsley sauce trickled over and a smidgeon of extra parsley.

Note:

A beef stomach may be thoroughly sliced with the useful resource of one's butcher. Otherwise, it could be wrapped in plastic wrap and saved inside the freezer for an hour or . This ought to make it less attackable and less difficult to slice.

Creamy Cauliflower Soup With Mustard Roasted Chickpeas

Ingredients (for four servings)

For the Soup:

1 small (300g) cauliflower head

2 celery stalks

1 small parsnip

1 parsley root

1 yellow onion

2 garlic cloves

1 tablespoon of tahini

3 cups of water

Pinch of sea salt

Freshly ground black pepper

half of teaspoon of caraway seeds

1 teaspoon of cumin powder

1 teaspoon of freshly squeezed lemon juice

For the Chickpeas:

1 can of cooked chickpeas

1 teaspoon of coconut oil

2 teaspoons of sugar-free mustard

half of teaspoon of cayenne pepper

1.   How to prepare

Begin through preheating the oven to one hundred 75°C/347°F.

Slice the cauliflower into florets, location right right into a bowl with salted water, and set aside for 5 minutes.

Rinse and drain the cauliflower, then steam for 10 minutes.

In a medium-sized soup pot, integrate the onions, parsley, celery stalks, and parsnip; fill with smooth water and boil over medium warmth.

Allow it to simmer on low warmness for 10 minutes.

Preparing the chickpeas:

Rinse the canned chickpeas, drain, and add to a baking tray.

Drizzle with oil, add mustard and cayenne, and toss to coat continuously.

Cook for 15 mins or until golden. Remove from the oven and set apart.

Transfer the liquid, vegetables, and steamed cauliflower into the blender, add tahini, garlic, salt, pepper, cumin, caraway, and lemon juice, and pulsate to benefit a creamy soup.

Pour into serving bowls, garnish with roasted chickpeas, and serve heat.

Hen's soup with double dumplings

Ingredients (for 4 servings)

Hen Soup:

1 whole chook

1 celery stick, chopped

2 leeks, thinly sliced

3 carrots, reduce into 1cm cubes

1 parsnip, reduce into 1cm cubes

1 teaspoon of black peppercorns

1/3 cup of parsley and wild garlic

Optional: Bay leaf, thyme, wild garlic, and parsley

Dumplings:

100g of butter

300g (2 cups) of simple flour

1 tablespoon of salt

three eggs

Meatballs:

300g of beef mince

2 slices of white bread, crust-a super deal a whole lot less

2 tablespoons of milk

1 egg

50g of butter

1 teaspoon of salt

half of of teaspoon of grated nutmeg

How to put together

For the stock:

Begin via setting the bird into a huge pan and consisting of enough water, making sure the fowl is completely submerged.

Let the bird boil over excessive warmth, then drain and rinse it underneath flowing water from the tap.

Put the hen right into a clean pan, and upload 4 liters of water or sufficient to cover the fowl. After that, allow it to simmer over medium warm temperature.

Add the bouquet garni, parsnip, celery, leek, carrots, and peppercorns. Reduce the warmth and prepare dinner on a low simmer for an hour. This lets in any impurities to upward push to the floor.

Take out the chook and set it apart for later use. Remove and discard the bouquet garni.

For the dumplings:

Bring 250ml (1 cup) water to a boil in a small pan.

Remove from the hearth after which includes the butter and stirring until melted.

Stir on the equal time as consisting of the flour and salt till there is a smooth consistency. Then whisk in the eggs one after the opposite until its properly blended.

Place in a bowl and allow to rest for twenty minutes.

To put together the meatballs:

Beat all the materials in a food processor till truly blended.

Mold the meatball and dough mixture into 2cm balls. Ensure you hold them apart.

Cook the meatballs and dumplings one after the opposite in a simmering, lightly salted water pan until they glide to the pinnacle.

Take them out of the pan with a slotted spoon. Set them apart.

Share the dumplings and meatballs in soup bowls first. Then add the vegetables and steaming soup.

To serve, garnish the meal with parsley and wild garlic.

Gluten-loose rugelach with cranberry port jam, chocolate, and walnuts

Ingredients (for four servings)

Cranberry Port Jam:

1 and 1/four cups of sparkling (or frozen) cranberries

half cup of sugar

half of of a vanilla bean, split lengthwise and scraped

1/three cup of ruby port

Cream Cheese Dough:

half of cup of candy white rice flour

1/four cup of millet flour

1/4 cup of gluten-unfastened oat flour

1/four cup of cornstarch

2 tablespoons of sugar

half of of teaspoon of xanthan gum

1/4 teaspoon of salt

6 tablespoons of cold, unsalted butter

8 tablespoons of cold cream cheese

Filling and Topping:

2/3 cup of walnut halves, gently toasted and cooled

2/3 cup of finely chopped chocolate

1 tablespoon of sugar

1/4 teaspoon of cinnamon

1 tablespoon of heavy cream (or milk or water)

1.   How to put together

Making the jam:

Combine the cranberries, sugar, vanilla pod, and scrapings in a small, heavy-bottomed pan. Allow it to boil over medium warm temperature, after which simmer for 10-15 mins over low heat till thick and chunky, stirring regularly to prevent burning.

Let the jam cool completely.

Making the dough:

In a meals processor bowl, combine the rice, millet, and oat flour with the cornstarch, sugar, xanthan gum, and salt.

Add the butter and cream cheese bits and method until the dough bureaucracy huge masses.

Place the dough on a piece of parchment paper and make certain it office work proper right into a hard log. Wrap the dough with each unique piece of parchment paper, then use a rolling pin to mildew the dough into a long and thin rectangle. With each few strokes of the pin, peel once more the pinnacle piece of parchment, area it once more on the dough, turn the dough and papers upside-down, peel lower back the modern-day top piece of paper, location it again on the dough, and continue. If the dough sticks to the paper, dirt it lightly with millet flour. If your rectangle is greater oval, you could trim the tough ends, stick them onto the corners, and hold rolling so one can form an fantastic rectangle.

Once the dough is rolled out, trim all the edges flat and instantly. Reserve the dough at cool room temperature at the same time as you prepare the fillings.

Preparing the fillings:

Pulsate the toasted and cooled walnuts in the food processor till finely chopped. Dump the walnuts into a bowl and wipe out the food processor.

Remove the vanilla pod from the chilled cranberry goop and add the goop to the meals processor.

For the puree smooth, add in three/four to at least one tbsp. Of sugar and cinnamon and stir, then set aside.

Assembling the rugelach:

Slide the rolled-out dough, even though on its parchment, onto a rimless cookie sheet for smooth coping with.

Thinly spread the cranberry jam over the dough, leaving a half of-inch border on each lengthy facets. Sprinkle the chocolate constantly over the jam, and sprinkle the ground walnuts over the chocolate. Use your fingers to pat everything down; the nuts and chocolate will adhere to the jam, making the rugelach less complex to roll.

Lift along the parchment's side and use it to roll up the rugelach as snugly as viable. It's ok if the dough cracks a hint. When the rugelach log is rolled, leave it seam-side down.

Chapter 5: Norwegian Porridge

Ingredients (for four servings)

Short Grain Rice:

This detail will make the lowest of the porridge. Short-grain rice is used thinking about that it's far fatter and stickier than ordinary rice.

Water:

Water is introduced to prepare dinner the rice.

Milk:

Milk will thicken the porridge, giving it a creamy texture. One can use plant-based totally milk which incorporates coconut milk or unsweetened oat milk; however, this might no longer hold the functionality to get as thick because the specific recipe intended.

Butter:

The use of butter offers the food richness and saltiness.

Honey:

Honey gives the porridge a bloomy satisfactory and a herbal sweetness. Ensure the honey used is preferred, as there are numerous flavors to be had.

Granulated Sugar:

Without any extra factors, sugar makes matters sweeter. It completes the dish and offers it a breakfast-like taste.

Kosher Salt:

Only a hint salt is wanted to stability out the splendor of the porridge. This ought to furthermore carry out more notes of taste from the opportunity elements.

Vanilla Extract:

A little vanilla permeates the dish with a fashionable caramel flavor and a lovable jasmine-like aroma.

Optional however Highly Recommended Toppings:

Cinnamon Powder:

A sprinkling of cinnamon affords spice and a clove-like taste for your breakfast bowl.

Dried Cranberries:

Dried cranberries will make the bowl of porridge fruit even as which includes greater texture and colour.

Butter:

This can be added on the pinnacle.

Brown sugar-roasted beef tenderloin.

Ingredients (for four servings)

1 boneless pork tenderloin

1 cup of dried figs, ideally chopped

1 cup of bourbon

2 heads of roasted garlic, with cloves squeezed out

8 ozof gorgonzola cheese, ideally crumbled

three tablespoons of smooth sage, chopped

2 tablespoons of brown sugar

1 teaspoon of dried herbs (such as thyme, rosemary, and oregano mixture)

1 teaspoon of salt

1 teaspoon of pepper

2 tablespoons of maple syrup

1 tablespoon of balsamic vinegar

How to put together

Begin via preheating the oven to 450°F.

Ensure you line the baking sheet or roasting pan with aluminum foil. Then observe the nonstick spray to it.

Put the beef on a cutting board, then slice it times to open it. Doing this could provide a whole lot of vicinity to art work with. Begin at the lowest of the beef and slice it vertically. Keep lowering to properly open up the pork.

Place the dried figs in a bowl, then warm temperature the bourbon in a pan over medium to low heat till it simmers. After that, pour the bourbon over the figs and permit them to soak for four to five minutes.

Generously spread the roasted garlic cloves at the inner of the red meat. Add the soaked and softened figs, crushed gorgonzola, and sage over the roasted garlic in that order.

Ensure you roll the tenderloin tightly and tie it collectively securely with kitchen wire. Then season the outdoor with herbs, salt, and pepper. Then rub the again with brown sugar.

Put the rolled-up tenderloin on a baking sheet or roasting pan. Make positive it roasts for thirty-5 to 40 minutes or until it is very well cooked on the inner (it need to have a take a look at approximately 140°C to a hundred 45°C). Also, make certain the red meat rest for 20 mins earlier than reducing.

Add two tablespoons of balsamic vinegar and maple syrup into the bourbon used to soak the figs. Reduce it via 1/2 in a pan over medium warmth. Drizzle this aggregate over the red meat proper before it is served.

HYGGE DRINK

Alewife

Ingredients (for two servings)

2 tsps. Of beetroot powder

three cups of milk of your choice

2 heaped tsp. Of Ginger or Ginger Marmalade

How to prepare

Begin through setting the marmalade and milk in a small pan over medium warm temperature. Cook till it's miles surely on the point of effervescent, but do no longer allow boiling.

Add a hint of boiled water to beetroot powder to make a paste in a small bowl. Mix with milk.

Pour into glasses and enjoy.

Note:

Beetroot powder or beetroot latte powder can be actually determined inside the health food phase of supermarkets.

Mulled wine

Ingredients (for 2 servings)

Wine: Make positive to choose out a bottle of wine that is not too pricey. Opt for a mid-variety bottle of dry pink or white wine. Fruity and complete-bodied wines like Zinfandel, Merlot, or Grenache work well for mulled wine as they may face up to heat, and their flavors are not clearly masked with the useful resource of the aromatics.

Brandy: It is traditional to spike your mulled wine with brandy. However, you may also use Cointreau, some other orange liqueur, or tawny port as alternatives.

Fresh oranges: You will want glowing oranges in your mulled wine. Slice a number of the oranges for mulling and use the rest for garnishing. If you choose an awful lot a whole lot less bitterness, you could peel the oranges in advance than simmering.

Cinnamon: Cinnamon sticks are quality for mulled wine. However, in case you do not have them, you can whisk in some floor cinnamon as an opportunity.

Mulling spices: Mulling spices can variety relying on the us. For a conventional aggregate, bear in mind the use of complete cloves and celebrity anise. You can also add some cardamom pods for brought flavor.

Sweetener: Adding sweetener is non-obligatory and may be adjusted to your taste. You can use sugar, maple syrup, or honey as natural sweeteners in your mulled wine.

How to put together

Begin by using way of combining factors. Put all materials in a pan and offer them a short stir.

Simmer over medium-excessive warm temperature till the wine nearly reaches boiling. It's vital no longer to allow it bubble in any way. The vaporisation temperature of alcohol is 172°F, so be cautious to make sure that the wine does not evaporate. Cover clearly, hold the heat on low, and permit the wine to boil lightly for fifteen minutes to three hours.

Using a brilliant mesh strainer to do away with and do away with the orange slices, cloves, cinnamon sticks, well-known individual anise, and ginger.

Stir the mulled wine and taste it; upload within the desired amount of greater sweetener if required.

Mulled wine is high-quality served warm in heatproof mugs. Garnish with toppings of your preference.

1.   Tibetan Tea or Butter Tea

Ingredients (for 2 servings)

2 pinches of Tea Leaves

Quarter cup Milk

Pinch of Salt

2 ½ cups of water

How to put together

The way for making Tibetan tea is simple. All one dreams is 8-10 minutes to make this tea.

Begin with the resource of boiling the water in a pan and then float the flame.

Throw the 2 pinches of tea within the water, hold to boil for a few minutes, after which separate the tea leaves.

Combine the tea, salt, butter, and milk in the blender and mix for 2-three mins.

Pour right into a cup and revel in.

Note:

The following aspect outcomes also can accompany Tibetan tea:

Caffeine: The caffeine content in butter tea is immoderate and may adversely have an effect at the body as soon as ate up in massive portions. Excessive intake of butter tea also can reason anxiety, sleep hassle, headaches, irritability, and stomach pain.

Cholesterol: Butter has some perfect fats and tremendous consequences on the frame. However, it nevertheless can reason some cardiovascular complications due to increases within the levels of cholesterol in your body.

Salt: Excessive indulgence can be unfavorable to our our our bodies. Adding too much salt to at least one's eating regimen can result in excessive blood strain. So, warning want to be achieved at the same time as making Tibetan tea to make certain the salt isn't always immoderate.

Slow Cooker Gingerbread Latte

Ingredients (for two servings)

eight cups entire milk.

1/four cup herbal maple syrup.

2 tablespoons packed brown sugar.

three tsp. Of ground ginger.

1 tsp. Of natural vanilla extract.

2 cinnamon sticks.

A pinch of cloves.

half tsp. Of sparkling ground nutmeg.

three and half of cups of strongly brewed coffee or coffee.

Whipped cream graham cracker crumbs, caramel sauce, and gingerbread cookies for garnish (non-compulsory).

How to prepare

Begin with the aid of manner of consisting of all substances to a huge gradual cooker.

Cook on low heat for approximately 3 hours or until heated via. Monitor to make sure it does not boil.

Turn the gradual cooker to a heat putting and put together dinner for some other 2 hours, stirring once in a while.

Dip rims of cups in caramel sauce after which in graham cracker crumbs. Top with easy whipped cream and caramel syrup or gingerbread cookies if p

referred. And Enjoy.

Sipping Caramel

Ingredients (for 2 servings)

1 cup of cream.

1/four cup of apple cider.

2 cups of sugar.

2 T of butter.

3 cups of skim milk.

Dash salt.

How to prepare

Begin by using using heating 1 cup of cream at the variety on low warmness; this have to be warmth but now not boiling.

Turn off the burner for cream and begin cooking 2 cups of sugar in a huge inventory pot.

Make extremely good to spread out the sugar calmly.

Turn on medium-excessive and constantly whisk after you see the sugar begin to soften.

Proceed to place on an oven mitt on your stirring hand.

Once all the sugar is melted, flip the warm temperature all the way down to the bottom setting; wait a couple of minutes in advance than slowly (on the identical time as stirring constantly) along with the nice and cozy apple cider.

Once the heavy boiling has subsided and the cider is jumbled together, do the identical with a bit of warmth cream.

Make positive you're constantly beating, and as quickly as the heavy boiling has lessened; throw within the 2 T of butter.

Continue to feature more warmness cream till it's miles prolonged past slowly.

After the butter has melted and all of the warmth cream has been jumbled collectively, slowly upload the three cups of skim milk.

Add the skim milk and apple cider so it does no longer reconstitute.

The sipping caramel should be very wealthy; you may be capable of similarly dilute it with milk to wholesome the taste.

You can keep the mixture after it has cooled and reheat it later. Enjoy.

Chapter 6: Body Clothing and Covering

Preamble

It's now not information that Hygge has taken the sector of interiors by means of typhoon. Many practitioners are eagerly updating their living areas to revel in the revel in as fast and as successfully as feasible. After all, with all of the chaotic mess going on every day in our world, it's far first-rate natural to want to move domestic to a fluffy paradise full of Blanche DuBois, suitable lighting fixtures, and a comfy surroundings.

Ideas at the lowest of Hygge style aren't that complex the least bit. It does no longer have to drain one's pocket or leave one in a nation in which they may revel in they've got underachieved or over-dressed. It embraces scarves, woolen socks, masses of monochrome colorations, and specific easy styling principles. That may moreover "Hygge-ify" one's fashion even as although staying proper to the obsessions of the season.

Basically, the sensation of being heat and relaxed sooner or later of the bloodless excursion season is valuable. One frequently desires to placed on what is going to make a formidable announcement about their character at the equal time as presenting protecting, warm temperature, and fashion. The best manner to gain consolation in wintry climate is thru manner of accepting the spirit of Hygge style whilst one gets dressed within the morning. Here, we're able to test some Hygge fashion options for actually every person searching for coziness, consolation, simplicity, and style to experience. These can also feature awesome gifts too.

Cozy Hygge Style Sweaters

Let's begin with cushty sweaters. Preferably for a few, sweaters that provide the feeling of Hygge are folks that give the sensation of one being wrapped up in a warm robe or blanket while they brunch up in style with friends. Here are some of the snug sweaters for each style and under:

1.   Let loose your wild issue with a certainly soft Snow Leopard Print Sweater.

2.   Look elegant and revel in comfortable with a extraordinary comfy, Chunky Knit Cardigan sweater.

3.   Wear a cowl neck Houndstooth Sweater from Nordstrom.

four.   Try a fuzzy V-Neck Sweater; this will be worn off the shoulder for a flirtier look.

5.   A Casual Turtleneck Pullover is first-rate for absolutely everyone and any occasion.

Warm Outerwear

Outerwear is a huge a part of our bloodless-climate apparel. Staying heat while searching one's extraordinary is important until one reaches there.

1.   Try a all of the time fashionable Wrap Wool Coat in checkered or stable shades. This can be paired with denims and boots for a

informal look or with a black skirt for a night day experience.

2.   A traditional Puffer Jacket is not first-rate fashionable however notably comfortable. A mid-duration model by using the use of Calvin Klein can positioned a smile on your face and that of your admirers.

3.   A traditional Trench Coat is extraordinary for any event, specially the stylish, prolonged, double-breasted types.

4.   Checkered Blanket Scarves hold you warmness and are available in severa adorable colorations to match custom seems.

5.   A Cozy Teddy Coat offers a lovely stability among the sensation of being tremendously snug and notably stylish.

Hygge Loungewear

In wintry climate, numerous humans's favored cold weather hobby is cuddling up next to the fireplace with a mug of heat chocolate whilst looking a film. This is due to the fact being warm and comfortable while one is indoors is just as important as while one is out and about. Here are some cozy loungewear and accessories to take into account:

1.   Perfect loungewear for lounging across the house is a Onesie. You can also get a first rate onesie from Amazon in a unmarried-of-a-type shade alternatives.

2.   Another object to encompass for your live-at-domestic fashion arsenal is the fluffy Fuzzy Slippers. This completes your cocoon of heat.

three. While on the couch, you can collect out for your warmth, Sherpa-style Throw Blanket to cuddle up with.

four.   A pair of at ease Jogger Pants can be worn from the residing room to the automobile to errands. They are quality for all-day luxurious and comfort.

5.   Another outfit is a comfortable group neck sweatshirt. This pulls the appearance

collectively to make any placing heat and a laugh.

Head-to-Toe Knits

Comfort is vital to Hygge, and knit clothing offers one of the maximum comforts for the body. Head-to-toe knitwear is not unusual nowadays and lovely; some can be easy ivory ensembles, even as others are decked out with dark beige fringe.

Comfy Socks

Socks are vital for preserving warmness and breeding that Hygge feeling on every occasion. A Fendi pair, worn with loafers, cropped trousers, and a bushy coat, is in truth elegant. You also can take a look at Dion Lee's fur-coated slippers.

Scarves

The preference of scarves ought to be in-between the big bulky scarves and the skinny ones. The sweet spot lies with selecting a quilted headband to fit your dress à l. A.

Chanel or knotting a sweater round your neck.

Layer is proper

You can't get enough layers. For the indoor Hygge practitioner, you could find out a layered look collectively with Gucci's sweatshirt-bomber-socks-leggings-pants outfit, which, it in order that occurs, synchronizes pleasantly with the decor.

Stick with the shade black.

Hygge flourishes on black and monochromes. There are a preference of style alternatives that completely blend in black with other monochrome solar sun sunglasses, which emerge as making ambitious style statements even as supplying masses-wished consolation.

Stay Warm when outdoor.

While carrying informal garb has advantages, it is although vital to stay heat and tone down the simplicity. A suitable midnight remedy is probably in reality one in each of Erdem's puffy jackets in sherbet tones or a cable-knit sweater from Dior.

Synchronize With Your Couch

The concept of hibernating interior throughout the cold winters paperwork the inspiration of hygge. Once inner, you will likely as nicely undergo in thoughts a way to coordinate your appearance along side your environment. Philosophy di Lorenzo Serafini's highly-priced couch and jewel-toned get dressed or à l. A. Rodebjer's matchy-matchy separates and painting.

Quality over amount

One of the matters about Danes is their pill fabric cabinet, having a mere large form of pleasant gadgets that circulate properly together, as contrasting to a protruding, mismatched series of garb. Copenhagen-based totally totally emblem, Woron offers remarkable basics. They produce vegan undies and style fundamentals that are absolutely Oeko-Tex Standard one hundred licensed.

HYGGE: TOGETHERNESS

1.   Preamble

Hygge really stands for cozying spherical together. Apparently, it's miles normal in Denmark to cluster collectively as massive households as soon as each week. This isn't always because of underdevelopment, where there isn't sufficient location and massive households are forced to percent a completely small vicinity. Parties and family gatherings offer numerous emotional resource for their attendees in techniques that pass neglected. There, pretty a few humans get to feel that they honestly belong. It can be a strong, satisfied haven to be snug, love, sing, dance, and so forth. For many, those sorts of gatherings are restoration.

This must no longer be muddled with abdication or sacrificing of all individual vicinity of information or want within the service of the larger unique or circle of relatives. In a Hygge, the character is also cherished; however, the knowledge is that with out the family contributors and guide of others, none people can be in truth content cloth as complete individuals. The journey must move from dependence to independence and then to interdependence.

A proper manner to see it is this: "When one replaces 'WE' with 'I,' even 'Illness' turns into 'Wellness.'" The phrase 'I' separates one's lips while pronouncing it, on the same time because the word 'we' truely brings one's lips collectively. These are clean techniques of seeing the significance of togetherness and contributors of the family with own family and buddies.

TEAMWORK IN HYGGE

In Denmark, kids are reinvigorated to paintings in teams pretty early in existence. They are taught to appearance out for the strengths and weaknesses in each unique and help perform the exceptional in each different. This teaches them essential thoughts of togetherness and encourages them to be high-quality group gamers. They study that by way of manner of the use of helping others, they inadvertently assist themselves, preserving them humble despite the fact that they turn out to be stars. They prepare dinner collectively, smooth up, and in large part discover techniques to experience each others' business enterprise.

Another manner of seeing this workout is through searching at how new mothers are supported in Denmark. To the cutting-edge mother, the indigenous midwife receives the statistics of all new mothers inside the community so she will be able to better control all the strain of having a ultra-contemporary toddler. Occasionally, those moms even go to each different. This offers a stable base of guide for brand spanking new moms as they will be capable of observe from the greater skilled ones; moreover they get assist on every occasion they require it. This does wonders to their feelings and our bodies in their maximum vital time.

So, right right here are some matters to be conscious for one to have Hygge togetherness:

1.   Begin through leaving the 'I' on your doorstep, together together with your cellphone, gadgets, and any and all physical self-attention. If you need to experience Hygge, then you definately need to be organized to bop and sing, no matter how ridiculous everything may probably sound or appearance; the concept is to be glad and make others glad.

2.   Live in the 2d. This technique no longer being held by way of way of the beyond and now not dreading the future. Instead, one is commonly encouraged to experience the present with buddies and own family.

How does one stay in the 2nd?

1.   Eliminate useless assets: Minimalism compels one to live inside the gift. Removing

objects associated with memories offers freedom from residing in the beyond.

2. Smile: Each day is complete of infinite possibilities. So, start it with a smile. Be on top of factors of your thoughts-set. Keep it great and expectant.

three. Cherish each 2d of these days: Take in as heaps of in recent times as feasible.; the marvels, resonances, aromas, sentiments, triumphs, and sorrows.

4. Forgive: Harboring resentment closer to a few other will only harm you. As the harm end up their fault, letting it have an impact for your mood nowadays is yours.

5. Think beyond vintage solutions to troubles: A lot of the day before today's solutions are no longer applicable solutions in recent times. Yesterday's answers aren't current day or tomorrow's answers.

6. Overcome addictions: These keep you hostage. They hold you from living a free life

and take away your focus from the instant. Let your self stay in the 2nd addiction-loose.

7.   Practice pre-framing. This is an influential device that helps you to form the idea technique of your mind about an occasion or hassle depend earlier than addressing it. An operative pre-body will permit you to align expectancies, cast off doubts, objections, and hesitations, and exhibit price-add and hassle-depend functionality.

8.   Have a laugh collectively. Each meeting and interest ought to be fun-filled. Do no longer be uptight and count on any shape of cheap bonding to arise. Make each interaction relaxed and thrilling via being engaged and collaborative, too.

9.   Confide and percent. This is a extraordinary tool for building togetherness. People who experience relaxed to confide with each other are effortlessly bonded and can proportion some aspect together. It is crucial, however, to appreciate the privacy of

others. Mutual appreciate is an crucial aspect within the widespread improvement of togetherness.

THE DANISH IDEA OF CHERISHING CHORES

The Danish concept of 'fællesskab' (community) is essentially the feeling of unison that comes from being in accord. There are kinds of fællesskab. One is the a laugh type that flows effects. This might be the sentiment that comes from gambling a amusing game or working together nicely with humans we get along side. We are painlessly a part of the group, and it's far amusing and comfortable. The one of a kind kind is the network sentiment we get from making an try to be a part of the agency even though we do now not typically want to be. This is known as a communal obligation. In Denmark, this is a vital a part of training and circle of relatives education and a wonderful lesson for the destiny.

Typically, one has to offer a few aspect to gather something from the fællesskab. It is possible which you cannot be getting all you need to your very personal way, so that you want to make a few concessions. It takes work to rely on every exceptional, and every so often, that could propose doing topics a hint in the route of your needs. One of the strategies to encourage fællesskab at home is thru doing chores together as a family. You can put together dinner collectively, smooth collectively or perhaps bake together.

Fællesskab is ready being more palms-on and collaborative in place of giving orders or doing everything on your very personal. It's a way of seeing everyday sports as an occasion as opposed to an impediment to spending time collectively. The right news is that the earlier you start, the extra it turns into a ordinary, and this could be placing your little one up for fulfillment in the end too.

One of the longest-strolling longitudinal research in data installation that one of the essential elements that add to expert accomplishment in lifestyles comes from doing chores as a infant. Children who often do chores are able to better address frustration, and now not on time pleasure, have higher self-self perception, and be extra responsible than people who do no longer do chores. So, in choice to giving an ultimatum for your toddler to clean up their room in any other case, or going to save and cook with the beneficial useful resource of yourself, see if you can discover a manner to art work collectively to create that feeling of 'fællesskab.' You might also additionally additionally find out that seeing your own family as a crew and treating them as such can be a tremendous way to bond ultimately.

HYGGE FOR FAMILY BONDING

Hygge is more of a intellectual idea than a bodily idea. The exercising works on one's psyche, lifting off weights of stress, negativity, and worries. It creates an surroundings that breeds being present in the suggest time and valuing precious instances spent together with own family and buddies. It is consciously putting try into giving up little portions of 1's self for the entire, inside the future at a time. It is giving up the "me time" for the "we time."

So, what should one do as a way to make stronger bonding, as a protracted manner as Hygge workout is worried?

1.   Make a decision on even as and the way extended you want to determine to hygge. This will beneficial useful resource you in being gift, due to the fact it is time restrained.

2.   Light candles as soon as you return interior. This can function a shape of Hygge sign for all dwellers inside the residence.

three. Make a addiction of turning off your devices and technological devices. This will decimate distractions.

four. Focus at the number one targets of Hygge- attempting to find coziness and tranquillity for your space. There may be splendid times to interest in your issues. So, loosen up collectively along with your pals and family, leaving normal stressors outdoor.

five.   Be intentional about showing gratitude for having possessions and people round.

6.   Be actively engaged. Sing and dance along facet your buddies and family. This has been confirmed to be exquisite for our nicely-being and is especially connecting. Once you circulate beyond the feelings of being stupid, you begin to appreciate how awesome it feels.

7.   Tell and reiterate humorous and horrifying memories from the past. This is a lovable manner to bond in the suggest time in a optimistic way.

Admittedly, it is able to be tasking occasionally to shut out the area for one's cherished ones; however, it's far an movement this is without a doubt simply worth it. One might also additionally bear in thoughts pausing and meditating for a couple of minutes on the the front door before taking walks into the house. This might probably assist refocus the thoughts and allow bypass of stressors simply so one may be present for their own family after they get domestic. What is crucial is the brilliant of time spent, no longer absolutely the amount. One may additionally have exquisite 20 mins to spare; make it count. Hygge may moreover sound like a walk in the park; but, it takes cognizance to rate this drama-free togetherness.

HYGGE FOR THE HOLIDAYS

Practicing Hygge isn't always a party pooper! One does no longer need to absolutely abandon their regular tactics of lifestyles and sink into some type of hiding inside the name of on the lookout for a snug, smooth, and glad lifestyles. This additionally applies to excursion seasons; Hygge can be protected into one's numerous holidays in case you want to initiate and hold the exercise of nurturing an surroundings of coziness, warmth, togetherness, and rest. In reality, for the reason that loads of pressure often accompanies the holiday season, Hygge is the suitable workout to imbibe with a purpose to reduce strain to a minimum.

Here are some Hygglige thoughts to assist make this demanding time a fulfilling and peaceful experience.

1.   Cut down a tree collectively as a family. Danes are identified to be into proper and herbal products. Many families there virtually chop it down bushes together from a farm. Such an hobby encourages teamwork and popular bonding. You should possibly select out to do some problem else, collectively with construct a small garden, choose up eggs, and so forth. All those should be natural and accomplished together. This can increase proper into a circle of relatives life-style fostering togetherness and delight. Any time this kind of circle of relatives way of existence is commemorated, you are making stronger the own family unit and be a part of coronary coronary coronary heart to heart. If you have

got a choice for plastic timber, that also may be finished. Simply positioned, positioned the tree in area and do the decorations together along a few Christmas song and baking cookies.

2. Light up the candles. Typically, there are a number of candles which is probably lit at Christmas anywhere from morning to night time time. This is in reality the prototypical look and experience of hygge at Christmas. They are in reality burning them generally of the day in houses and teashops. Most oldsters have a calendar candle, that is typically blown out at breakfast to suggest within the destiny has surpassed in the direction of Christmas. This is sincerely relaxed.

3. Hold palms, and sing across the tree. This is a adorable hygge culture. It is truly hyggelige to mild the candles on the Christmas tree. Everyone can then dance in the course of the Christmas tree, preserving palms and creating a music Christmas songs together earlier than taking off offers. This is

usually a amusing exercise for children, in spite of the reality that they ought to live up for their gadgets.

4.   Do a few baking and revel in lots of video video video games. Hygge is all approximately being present and playing time collectively. When Danes are all collectively all through the holidays, they commonly play many video games with the circle of relatives. Playing video games is a exceptional way to be present collectively inside the advise time. Also, baking modified into certainly taken into consideration considered one of their many practices; they typically bake many specific cookies collectively, with the children being considerably worried. Again, group strive is important in Hygge at Christmas. Everyone is aware that they assist out, selling a comfortable surroundings.

Chapter 7: Outdoor Practice

1.   Hygge and the notable outside

Hygge may be practiced out of doors. It isn't an particular indoor exercise. Getting the manner to do this can extensively enhance one's existence whilst far from home specifically and of their existence in current-day.

There are not any rubrics to pursuing Hygge dwelling in a single's outdoor recreations. However, if one is interested in taking up all of the warm temperature and coziness that the cooler weather has to offer, here is a list to help hatch that deeply preferred environment:

Rise early and opt for a dawn picnic

Begin through putting your alarm for an hour earlier than dawn, % a flask of espresso and your chosen baked pastries, take a cosy outside blanket, and visit a local park to look at the dawn. If you can discover a friend to return lower again along for the journey, that would be even lovelier. The feeling you may get from this revel in may be exceptional described as being next to none.

Build and feature fun with a patio hearth.

If you stay in a domestic in which you have were given an outdoor patio and might experience outside fires internal the hearth pit, then you have to take the a exquisite deal-wished step and experience each minute of it. You do no longer even need to make hundreds of a determination as it receives dark earlier inside the iciness months. So, pass in advance and slight a fireplace, invite your parents and buddies over to capture up, and make installed a few fun sports at the same time as savoring the outside.

Make a heat drink to enjoy outside.

There are numerous Hygge beverages that you may make, so why forestall at espresso or tea? You can revel in a special wintry weather warmer in a flask even as ambling across the out of doors or community.

Create a watercolor paint tin and use it outdoor.

Make a small pocket watercolor set to % on your rucksack for your subsequent outdoor experience. The idea right right here is set making art and taking time to realize and seize the magic of the outdoor.

Spend on cushty wool socks.

Darn Tough socks are designed in Vermont and include an unrestricted lifetime guarantee. They are synthetic with merino wool, are available in adorable sun sunglasses, and are the coziest problem to cover one's toes.

Hang outdoor string lighting fixtures inside the out of doors.

The evenings in the month of November are usually dark and from time to time lackluster. You can warmness subjects up with a string of fairy lighting. Dangle them near the decrease back door, at the porch, or round a tree that you'll be capable of see from the kitchen window. Solar string lighting fixtures are great for this considering the fact that one could not must plug them in, and they'll come on routinely at the same time as it gets dark. These sun string lighting are perfect for hygge residing outside.

Try stargazing

Once sunlight hours monetary financial savings time starts, the solar will start putting in the overdue afternoon. Instead of being blue over the darkness, clasp it with a stargazing escapade. Even despite the fact that the celebrities are adorable to test on any smooth nighttime, one might also need to test out the Taurids Meteor Shower in November, that is high-quality visible between the fifth and 12th.

Practice outdoor yoga out of doors.

Even if one already has a normal yoga exercise or has never tried it previously, schooling outdoor will assist in connecting with the natural worldwide on the equal time as bringing in a chunk of a task to at least one's workout. One can get some brilliant out of doors yoga poses from Yoga journals, books, or on line to assist them get started out out. Even a yoga mat is completely optionally to be had.

Attempt Letterboxing

Letterboxing is a type of out of doors treasure hunt. But no longer like its sister game-Geocaching, one does not need a GPS to move Letterboxing. Letterboxers use hints to search for their treasure, typically hidden in a natural spot. Discoverers make an inscription of the letterbox's stamp of their private logbook and go away an inscription in their personal stamp within the letterbox's logbook. It is a amusing workout.

Attempt a taking walks meditation.

Walking is one of the most common undertakings in regular life, and strolling meditation can be a commanding and frightening workout to beneficial resource one in bringing mindfulness into their each day existence. Walking meditation may be as modest as heedfully totaling one's steps as one walks and takes in truth minutes every day.

Fashion a candle lantern and moderate it outdoor.

There are countless DIY candle lantern mind to be had. You may want to lead them to out of prolonged-lasting embroidery foil, vintage tin cans, and glass jars. Whatever you have got got handy, flip that trash into treasure.

Stopover at a neighborhood farm

There isn't whatever like a day on the farm to position one in touch with their roots, whether or not or no longer following the each day sequences of livestock or the recurrent cycles of neighborhood produce.

Go cabin tenting

Regardless of in which one lives- in the metropolis, the outskirts, or the agricultural geographical region, you may be capable of normally benefit from a night time time time or a weekend away. One can positioned within the attempt and find out rustic cabins, tree houses, or yurts that encompass all topics hygge. Box the naked requirements for one's enjoy and be prepared to in truth be.

Go for a walk with a pal.

This is simple. Make plans to entice up with a chum on a walk round one's neighborhood or neighborhood park.

Take hold of your binoculars and watch the birds.

There is something extremely satiating about looking the birds that live near one's home. It is an outstanding way to benefit an records of herbal international and ecology. One could not want to be an professional to experience fowl searching, and it's far specifically fun to do with children.

Create a suet fowl circlet and cling it on your backyard for feathered buddies

A lot of birds love suet feeders, specially while the bloodless weather comes spherical. As an opportunity to a shop-offered suet feeder, it is straightforward to fashion an elegant suet wreath. It's a vacation decoration that birds experience.

Read your favourite e-book in a hammock.

Lazing within the hammock with one's preferred e-book isn't handiest for lazy summer time weekends. Pack up and head out of doors for a bit me time among your preferred wooden.

Spend on a few wintry climate woolens.

Wool wicks moisture away from one's pores and skin; it is able to absorb about 30% of its weight in water with out feeling wet and may adjust one's body temperature, retaining it cool inside the summer season and heat in the wintry climate. One's outdoor escapades is probably an awful lot more exciting with a few woolens to keep them relaxed. Invest in a

Merino base layer, some relaxed pullovers, and some wool mittens.

Ditch the GPS and opt for a pressure for your terrific pal

Take a brief avenue trip without a terminus in thoughts. Reconnoiter back roads, revel in the surroundings, and do not spark off the GPS until it's time to go home.

Go for your chosen outdoor spot and write on your mag

Having a favourite outdoor spot may be beneficial. This spot can be used as your stable area. Visit the spot, sit down down quite really, and spend fifteen minutes writing for your magazine.

Play a endeavor of tag or cowl-and-are searching for with a few pals

You can venture your spouse, kids, or pals to a sport of tag or cover-and-are looking for. This may be fun, deepening your connections.

Plant spring bulbs

It may additionally moreover appear dull now, however spring may be right right here earlier than we are privy to it. You can plant spring bulbs like daffodils, tulips, or hyacinths. Find a naked patch of soil, drop within the bulbs, water methodically, and forget about approximately them until spring.

Paddle a canoe or a kayak.

Pick a sunny day and opt for a overdue fall paddle. This is an splendid out of doors interest. You interact with nature, water, and the high-quality smells that accompany them.

Chapter 8: The Workplace

Bearing in mind the pressures that hundreds of human beings are dealing with within the place of work, we all have to make do with a hint extra aid balancing intellectual health and cutting-edge properly-being. Here are five strategies to permeate a bit of hygge into the workspace, wherever that might be proper now.

Connect with others

Hygge is prepared community and bringing people collectively. Grabbing a virtual lunch with co-employees or Face Timing with a cherished you may honestly flow into a protracted way in lifting moods these days. You have to even send a card or be aware inside the mail to feel that experience of connection. Be careful, although, now not to be distracted from surely strolling.

Exercise mindfulness

Take a two-minute damage frequently to popularity first-rate on respiration or do a little moderate stretching at your table. There are quite a few mindfulness apps to assist guide the technique. Survey reviews have set up that about 26% of U.S. Offices provide meditation/mindfulness education.

Sip a few tea or Hygge beverage.

For instantaneous Hygge, just upload a heat, cozy beverage together with warm chocolate, tea, or espresso. The fact is over half of of (sixty 4%) of U.S. Places of labor offer a coffee provider.

Decorate your workspace with a few love.

Decorate with a few pictures of humans and things you like, art work that makes you satisfied, desired pens, a plant or , or maybe a small accent lamp if vicinity lets in. Some decluttering can useful resource in taking component in a relaxed, at ease location to be industrious anywhere your workspace might be.

Be top notch

Company and sociability are essential additives of Hygge. Think of techniques you could make art work amusing on your coworkers, even though it is sincerely. Remember a coworker's birthday or anniversary, send them a fruit basket, or assist them after they need it. This will cheer them up, and it will raise you as well.

HYGGE WITH A BUDGET

WHERE DOES ONE BEGIN?

As said previously, Hygge is a country of mind; it's miles the sensation of coziness, comfort in existence, and in which and the manner one is at present. Hygge is not about buying plenty of posh subjects to make one feel better. In truth, it is pretty the other. It is prepared finding contentment in small ordinary sorts of stuff. How can one be relaxed and have Hygge on your everyday lifestyles with out spending too much or going over one's charge range?

Music

Begin by way of manner of employing your preferred tune in the ancient past while you paintings, do chores, or bake. You can also even permit the song play at the same time as sitting and absorbing the environment. Some people ought to choose listening to a podcast or an audiobook. Whatever the case, it is important to get what works for you.

Book

Reading may be therapeutic. Studies have indicated, however, that studying an real ebook rather than a virtual one is more fun and higher for the eyes. So, strive reading a e-book; spend time in your favored spot, reading and reflecting.

Tea Or Coffee

Tea, further to coffee, are of the least high-priced liquids to shop for and eat. They provide refreshments on the same time as taken as one cuddles underneath the blanket at the equal time as taking note of music or studying a book.

Now, one might also have to buy special topics to assist decorate the enjoy. Things consisting of candles, decorations, fluffy pillows, comfortable blankets, and an array of clean however monochrome collections of wears, mufflers, socks, and so on are all desired. However, there can be no need to interrupt the economic institution. Nothing extravagant is wanted in any example.

OTHER THINGS TO HAVE HANDY

Hygge is ready simplicity and contentment. It is ready playing and embracing lifestyles and happiness. If you want to, you may add a number of the following on your Hygge mixture:

Essential Oils

Essential oils in reality aid one's well-being and being cushty. They are to be had numerous types and paperwork. Choose the ones which you like and stick with them. Make sure to check the smell earlier than you buy any.

Dinner With Friends

Hygge is not all approximately being on my own but spending time with cherished ones and sharing moments of pride, and being cushty with each wonderful. It is prepared social coziness, in which one stocks fun and a bit with others. So, gain out to a chum and installation your subsequent dinner date.

Comfortable Clothing

Having comfortable apparel makes you comfortable collectively along side your surroundings. By wearing snug clothes, one is certainly doing Hygge with out questioning they will be.

HYGGE PRACTICE IN CERTAIN SEASONS

WAYS TO PRACTICE HYGGE IN A WARM CLIMATE

Wear apparel crafted from herbal-fiber

Clothing crafted from natural, breathable fibers is maximum comfortable on the identical time because the temperature is heat. Two first rate examples are cotton and linen. When one options clothing for Hygge in a warm temperature climate, the technique for gaining comfort lies within the natural material's knack for breathing.

Employ the use of gentle textures.

Wear loose, flowing garments to exercise Hygge on the same time because the temperatures are warmness. Wrap a mild-weight blanket or throw it over the sofa to cover up and experience at ease with out getting too warm. Employ greater gentle textures to the house, together with toss pillows and consuming chair cushions.

Ba amongst pals and circle of relatives

The Danish idea of Hygge is closely associated with great gatherings. Such gatherings want to be easy-going, casual, and spontaneous. Even while the climate is warm temperature, we are able to experience the spirit of Hygge with the resource of getting together with those we like.

Get involved in unplanned, laid-lower back sports.

Think of Hygge as a body of mind for each day sports activities. In warmness temperatures, the ones is probably open-air activities like taking a stroll, using a motorcycle, or walking thru a park. Or, they might be indoor interests, like running on a jigsaw puzzle, analyzing, or delighting in a communique with someone you want.

Adopt simplistic dwelling

Simplistic dwelling is a applicable key to Hygge, regardless of what one is doing-getting prepared a meal, getting kitted out, or scheduling a assembly. There's no want for conventionalism or stressful conditions within the pursuit of Hygge.

Indulge in relaxation

Hygge encourages its practitioners to continuously gradual down and lighten up. It is about pausing and taking a breather. Life these days is rapid-paced. One needs to slow down and loosen up.

Go out on a picnic

In warmth climates, the solstice warmth and humidity make eating outdoors a spiteful experience. Nevertheless, ingesting outside is a pleasant enjoy in the fall, wintry weather, and spring seasons. Practice Hygge with the useful resource of occurring a picnic, consuming in the outdoor vicinity of a restaurant, or genuinely relishing a meal within the out of doors. Regardless of the temperature, you will be able to pick comfortable and comfortable options.

Make your home a cushty sanctuary.

Once your living location is spotless and uncluttered, it will become much less complicated to workout Hygge. Light a few aromatic candles or prompt a diffuser to emit critical oils into the air. Toss some mild pillows on the sofa and add a mild-weight throw. Before prolonged, you may be training hygge in your personal peaceable, warm weather area.

FORMULATING A WEEKEND OF HYGGE

A WEEKEND ROUTINE FOR HYGGE

A weekend regular is a manner to stop one's weekends from really fizzling out inside the vapor of chores and trap-up which stand inside the manner of doing the fun stuff or embarking on large duties that would preserve deeper importance. Without a weekend ordinary, it might be not feasible to workout Hygge. This is because of the reality the Hygge exercising is time-eating and could commonly require planning. If one does not make plans, subjects may additionally grow to be being overwhelming ultimately.

WHAT A WEEKEND ROUTINE IS NOT

A weekend recurring ought to not be a few shape of tightly scheduled, delight-killing tactic to manipulate your weekend. Inasmuch as it isn't always meant to feature to at the least one's frustration, it isn't always intended to choke the life out of Hygge either, via stress, compulsion, anxiety inducement, and so on. If it creates even extra strain, then it has lost its charge even before it receives done.

So, developing a weekend ordinary targets to get via the vital jobs whilst making time for rest and a laugh. It need to generally purpose a stability in downtime, family time, and being productive with one's time.

THE BENEFITS OF A WEEKEND ROUTINE

For numerous humans, the weekend takes place to be their downtime, family time, or a laugh time. It should permit one to lighten up after a busy week at the equal time as placing one up for a a success week in advance. A weekend habitual can assist with this with the resource of helping one in getting via the stuff they need to do while giving them lower lower back the time to carry out a touch issue they need. Creating a notable weekend ordinary in vicinity will:

1.	Make positive all of the vital obligations get completed

2.	Leave one extra organized for the week beforehand

3.	Give one the time to do the a laugh stuff they want to do

4.	Free up time to hobby on any weekend obligations you have been making plans

5.	Make one's weekends calmer and additional exciting

6.	Give one once more Sunday evenings as a time to lighten up or do an interest

7.	Make the start of the modern-day week much less tough

8.	Make the weekends experience longer as one is not chasing their tail and beginning to recollect subsequent week early on Sunday.

Chapter 9: How to Make a Weekend Routine

1.   The first step is to listing down duties you want to accomplish inside the course of the weekend. This have to range from own family chores together with laundry and cleaning to out of doors sports activities consisting of purchasing. Most importantly, it need to additionally encompass the property you need to get set for Monday and the upcoming week. Generally, this could no longer exchange weekly, so it'll shape the mainstay of your normal weekend routine.

2.   Then on the start of each weekend, if in any respect viable, with a pitcher of wine as you lighten up on Friday night time, sit down and appraise what Hygge activities are taking location that weekend. It might be playing sports activities sports, youngsters' instructions, birthday events, circle of relatives sports, meeting up with friends, and so forth. Get them all into the calendar early after which plan everything else spherical them.

three. Once all the scheduled devices you need to do are logged in, you may start to work on what you'll likely need to do. These might be spending time with own family, taking place an day ride, doing a interest, cocktail hour, date night time time, a own family recreation or movie night time, and so on.

4.   There might be no want to have a strict timetable which you observe to the minute, as this is not the purpose right here. It is commonly enough to really allocate matters to durations, at the side of Saturday afternoon, in vicinity of a particular time. It additionally may be absolutely useful to set a motive for every day of the weekend. This might possibly exchange from week to week. However, the greater you get used to questioning this manner, the much less complex it will become.

5.   Check your plan and make certain the routine is not over-booked. Don't fill up your weekends with too many plans, outings, and

sports. You'll virtually end up exhausted and no longer feeling refreshed and prepared for next week.

TIPS FOR YOUR WEEKEND ROUTINE

1.   Figure out what you actually need from your weekends and use the normal that will help you in accomplishing it. Deliberately making plans out your weekends can move an prolonged way to helping you in getting the weekend time you need.

2.   You can rearrange your assignment finally of the week, shifting some duties from being finished at the weekday to the weekend and vice versa. As a end result, you can manage your obligations in order of priority at some level within the week, and some time desk might be uncluttered.

3.   Involve the rest of the family. It takes a group attempt to perform any set of plans in a household. When anybody is worried, the time spent on each chore is lessen

appreciably at the same time as the bond amongst parents is strengthened.

four. Don't worry if the plan is going off-track. Weekends are mainly for gambling your self, so in case you get a closing-minute invitation to a grill, then say yes with the guilt-free information that your weekend ordinary has taken care of numerous the weekend jobs for you.

five. A new habitual, just like a contemporary exercise, takes time to settle in. Unavoidably, the primary few weeks might also have knocks, and you can need to alter the plan to suit you and your family better. That's high-quality in choice to unwanted. Soon, you could have a weekend habitual it is simple, controllable, and aids with stress in vicinity of producing it.

Chapter 10: Traditional Scandinavian Dishes

Scandinavian cuisine is wealthy in records and traditions, with each United States of America of the United States within the vicinity having its very very own unique culinary historic beyond. The traditional dishes of Scandinavia are diagnosed for their simplicity, reliance on network components, and emphasis on preserving meals for the prolonged, harsh winters. Let's find out the assessment of conventional Scandinavian dishes in this newsletter.

Smorgasbord: A Culinary Extravaganza

One iconic hassle of Scandinavian delicacies is the smorgasbord, a buffet-style meal that showcases a huge kind of dishes the phrase "smorgasbord" itself way "sandwich table" in Swedish. It usually includes a series of open-faced sandwiches, cold cuts, pickled herring, smoked fish, meatballs, salads, and numerous condiments.

The smorgasbord isn't best a ceremonial dinner for the taste buds however additionally a seen delight. It reflects the Scandinavian technique to food, specializing in freshness, simplicity, and presentation. The abundance of dishes allows visitors to pick out their favorites and encourages a social and convivial consuming enjoy.

A Celebration of Seafood

Given their proximity to the ocean, it's miles no surprise that seafood performs a prominent function in conventional Scandinavian cuisine. Fish which incorporates salmon, herring, cod, and trout are normally applied in hundreds of arrangements. One famous Scandinavian dish is gravlax, this is raw salmon cured in a mixture of salt, sugar, and dill. The cured salmon is thinly sliced and served with mustard sauce, dill, and conventional crispbread.

Pickled herring is another preferred Scandinavian seafood delicacy. It is frequently served with onions, dill, and bitter cream, and is a staple on the smorgasbord. The herring is commonly cured in a mixture of vinegar, sugar, and spices, ensuing in a tangy and slightly candy flavor.

Rooted in Nature: Foraging and Wild Ingredients

Scandinavian delicacies has a sturdy connection to nature, and foraging performs a large function in traditional dishes. The large forests and pristine landscapes provide an abundance of untamed materials which is probably incredibly valued in Scandinavian cooking.

One such thing is the lingonberry, a small tart berry that grows in the wild. Lingonberries are implemented in numerous strategies, from making jams and sauces to accompanying meat dishes like Swedish meatballs. Their bright crimson colour provides a colourful contact to the plate.

Another foraged element is the chanterelle mushroom. These golden-hued mushrooms are prized for his or her touchy flavor and are regularly sautéed with butter and served as a aspect dish or included into stews and soups.

Preserving the Harvest: Curing, Smoking, and Fermenting

Preservation techniques are essential to traditional Scandinavian cooking, as they allow the locals to experience their favourite components during the three hundred and sixty five days. Curing, smoking, and fermenting are not unusual strategies used to keep meals.

Gravlax, said earlier, is a top instance of curing. By combining salt, sugar, and dill, the salmon is preserved and develops a totally particular taste profile. Similarly, smoking is appreciably used for maintaining fish, mainly salmon and herring. The smoking way no longer most effective imparts a outstanding smoky flavor but furthermore extends the shelf life of the fish.

Fermentation is any other protection technique that provides intensity and complexity to Scandinavian dishes. Fermented elements like sauerkraut, pickles, and diverse dairy merchandise are usually enjoyed. For example, lutefisk, a traditional dish made from dried and cured whitefish, is soaked in water and lye to soften it earlier than cooking. The lye answer gives the fish a gelatinous texture and a very specific taste.

Famous Scandinavian Recipes and Their Secrets

Scandinavian delicacies is renowned for its iconic recipes which have stood the test of time. Let's discover some famous dishes and the secrets and techniques and strategies at the back of their achievement.

1. Swedish Meatballs

Swedish meatballs, or "köttbullar," are a cherished Scandinavian dish that has obtained international fame. These mild and flavorful meatballs are historically made from a combination of floor beef and red meat, blended with breadcrumbs, onions, and spices inclusive of allspice and nutmeg. The thriller to their melt-in-your-mouth texture lies within the addition of cream or milk to the aggregate. The meatballs are generally served with creamy gravy and lingonberry sauce, followed via potatoes or noodles.

2. Norwegian Fårikål

Fårikål is a hearty and comforting Norwegian dish that holds a special area within the hearts of Norwegians. It is a easy stew made with lamb meat and cabbage, flavored with black peppercorns and salt. The dish is sluggish-cooked, permitting the flavors to meld collectively and the meat to come to be easy and succulent. Fårikål is historically cherished in the end of the fall months, and it's miles often served with boiled potatoes and lingonberry jam.

3. Danish Smørrebrød

Smørrebrød is an iconic Danish open-faced sandwich that exemplifies the Scandinavian love for rye bread and progressive toppings. The bread is generally dense and hearty, topped with a number of additives which encompass pickled herring, smoked salmon, liver pâté, roast beef, and severa spreads like remoulade or mayonnaise. The key to a scrumptious smørrebrød lies within the stability of flavors and the suave association of toppings. It is a culinary masterpiece that showcases every flavor and seen attraction.

four. Finnish Karjalanpiirakka

Karjalanpiirakka, also referred to as Karelian pasties, is a traditional Finnish dish that originated within the place of Karelia. These small pastries are made from a rye flour dough and complete of a mixture of rice and butter. They are usually cherished as a savory snack, regularly crowned with a slice of butter and served with egg butter or some of conventional Finnish cheese. Karjalanpiirakka is a favored staple of Finnish cuisine, and its delicate stability of flavors and textures makes it a real delight.

five. Icelandic Hangikjöt

Hangikjöt is a traditional Icelandic dish that showcases the united states's unique approach of smoking meat. It is historically crafted from lamb that has been cured, smoked, after which boiled or roasted. The smoking machine infuses the beef with a splendid smoky flavor, whilst the slow cooking guarantees tenderness. Hangikjöt is regularly served with boiled potatoes, white sauce, and peas, growing a fulfilling and comforting meal.

Chapter 11: Scandinavian Design

The Principles of Scandinavian Design

Scandinavian layout has received international reputation for its simplicity, functionality, and undying beauty. Rooted inside the countries of Denmark, Sweden, and Norway, this format aesthetic has end up synonymous with easy strains, minimalism, and natural materials. The ideas of Scandinavian format now not exceptional popularity on aesthetics however additionally emphasize practicality and the use of slight to create harmonious dwelling areas. In this article, we're capable of delve into the center mind that define Scandinavian layout.

Simplicity and Minimalism

At the coronary heart of Scandinavian layout lies the idea of simplicity and minimalism. Scandinavian designers attempt to create regions which is probably uncluttered, with a focal point on critical factors. This format philosophy embraces the idea of "a fantastic deal less is extra." By putting off vain ornamentation and maintaining best the critical elements, Scandinavian layout achieves a experience of calm and tranquility. Clean lines, uncluttered areas, and a impartial color palette are key additives of this format method.

Functionality and Practicality

Scandinavian format locations a sturdy emphasis on capability and practicality. Each piece of furniture or accessory is carefully designed to serve a cause and meet the desires of the purchaser. The interest is on developing designs that are not simplest aesthetically attractive but additionally especially realistic. Furniture frequently functions modular factors, multifunctional designs, and innovative storage solutions. Scandinavian designers purpose to beautify the man or woman's regular lifestyles with the aid of the use of developing objects which can be adorable, durable, and serve a practical motive.

Natural Materials and Textures

Another awesome characteristic of Scandinavian format is the usage of natural materials and textures. Wood, specifically light-colored woods which includes pine and birch, is a hallmark of Scandinavian interiors. These materials deliver warm temperature, character, and a enjoy of nature into the space. The grain and texture of the timber are regularly celebrated, with furniture and flooring showcasing their herbal beauty. Other substances usually placed in Scandinavian layout include leather-based, wool, linen, and herbal fibers. These substances create a tactile enjoy and make contributions to the general comfy and inviting environment.

Light and Airiness

Scandinavian international locations experience prolonged, dark winters, that have inspired the importance of mild in format. Maximizing herbal slight and developing extremely good, airy areas is a crucial element of Scandinavian format. Large home home windows, skylights, and open floor plans are common abilties in Scandinavian interiors, allowing sufficient herbal mild to flood the space. Light-colored partitions, light-toned furniture, and strategically placed mirrors are used to mirror and extend the mild, making rooms appear more spacious and welcoming.

Harmonious Color Palette

Scandinavian design commonly favors a harmonious and constrained shade palette. White and diverse sun shades of grey function a backdrop, allowing the natural substances and textures to take middle level. Soft, muted colors which includes slight blues, pastel pinks, and light earthy tones also are used to characteristic subtle touches of color. The cause of this subdued color palette is to create a revel in of serenity and stability inside the vicinity, while also enhancing the herbal mild.

Timelessness and Longevity

Scandinavian format is famend for its timelessness and sturdiness. The attention on simplicity, functionality, and incredible craftsmanship ensures that Scandinavian portions stand the take a look at of time each aesthetically and structurally. The easy lines and minimalistic aesthetic cross past passing traits, making Scandinavian layout quantities a profitable investment. This layout philosophy encourages sustainability with the resource of selling long lasting, nicely-crafted gadgets that may be cherished for destiny years.

Scandinavian Nature

Introduction to the Breathtaking Landscapes of Scandinavia

Scandinavia is renowned for its breathtaking landscapes that captivate the creativeness and leave site visitors in awe. This place, consisting of Norway, Sweden, Denmark, Finland, and Iceland, offers a numerous range of natural splendor, from majestic fjords and towering mountains to pristine forests and shimmering lakes. Let us embark on a journey via the captivating landscapes of Scandinavia, exploring the right abilties that make this region a haven for nature lovers.

Scandinavia is domestic to a number of the maximum stunning fjords inside the global. Fjords are prolonged, slender inlets carved via glaciers at some stage in the Ice Age. The Norwegian fjords, in particular, are famous for his or her dramatic cliffs and deep blue waters that replicate the surrounding mountains. One of the most iconic fjords is the Geirangerfjord, a UNESCO World Heritage Site. Its cascading waterfalls, sheer rock partitions, and pricey greenery create a surreal environment that transports site website traffic into a international of natural splendor.

Mountains additionally play a prominent function in shaping Scandinavia's landscapes. The Scandinavian Mountain Range, additionally referred to as the Scandes, stretches across Norway, Sweden, and a small part of Finland. These mountains provide breathtaking vistas and possibilities for out of doors sports sports such as hiking, snowboarding, and natural global spotting. The highest peak, Galdhøpiggen, reaches an fantastic height of ,469 meters, presenting panoramic views that amplify for miles. In Sweden, the Abisko National Park offers a enchanting alpine panorama with snow-capped peaks, glaciers, and crystal-clean lakes.

The place's forests are every different herbal treasure. Scandinavia is home to widespread expanses of lush green forests, which are not simplest visually cute but moreover harbor a wealthy biodiversity. The Taiga forests, observed in northern Scandinavia, are the most important contiguous forested region in Europe. These forests are characterized through a tapestry of coniferous wood, which incorporates spruce, pine, and birch. Walking thru these forests, one can also need to revel in a experience of tranquility, due to the reality the dense foliage gives a serene environment and shelters an array of natural international.

Now, allow's dive into the flora and fauna precise to Scandinavia. The region's lengthy, bloodless winters and relatively quick summers have not unusual the plant and animal lifestyles, ensuing in some of species which have adapted to the ones tough situations. Scandinavia boasts an notable form of wildflowers that bloom inside the direction of the summer season, consisting of colorful shades to the landscapes. The Arctic poppy, Lapland rosebay, and woman's slipper orchid are only some examples of the tremendous vegetation that may be observed in this vicinity.

When it involves fauna, Scandinavia is domestic to severa iconic animals. In the Arctic tundra of Svalbard, polar bears reign very high-quality, at the same time as reindeer roam the big barren region of Lapland. The Scandinavian brown undergo, lynx, and wolverine may be located in the dense forests, at the same time as beavers build their dams in the area's waterways. Bird lovers might be extraordinarily comfortable through manner of the sight of majestic sea eagles soaring via the skies, and the haunting name of the loons echoing at some stage in the tranquil lakes.

As we venture in addition into Scandinavia, we discover hidden gems and herbal wonders which might be off the overwhelmed path. From secluded waterfalls nestled in deep valleys to mystical caves carved via historical rivers, the place is entire of surprises organized to be determined. One such gem is the Lofoten Islands in Norway. These far off islands boast dramatic cliffs, white sandy seashores, and colourful fishing villages, developing a picturesque setting that attracts photographers and nature enthusiasts alike. The unique mixture of rugged mountains, pristine waters, and captivating purple and yellow cottages make the Lofoten Islands an idyllic holiday spot.

Scandinavia is likewise home to severa natural wonders that leave traffic in awe of the Earth's geological marvels. One such surprise is Iceland's well-known Golden Circle. This famous traveller direction encompasses 3 lovely points of interest: the powerful Gullfoss waterfall, the Geysir geothermal vicinity with its erupting heat springs, and the historical Þingvellir National Park, wherein website online visitors can walk between the Eurasian and North American tectonic plates.

Another natural marvel properly really worth exploring is the Midnight Sun phenomenon. During the summer season months in northern Scandinavia, the sun does not absolutely set, casting a perpetual golden glow over the landscapes. This surreal experience lets in for prolonged daytime, supplying good enough time to discover and understand the beauty of the vicinity.

For the ones in search of a real barren area experience, the Lapland vicinity gives a paranormal get away. Located inside the direction of Finland, Sweden, Norway, and Russia, Lapland is known for its huge barren location, snow-blanketed landscapes, and the possibility to witness the spell binding Northern Lights. In wintry climate, website online site visitors can enjoy sports activities activities together with dog sledding, snowmobiling, or maybe spending a night time time in an ice lodge.

Scandinavia's archipelagos are a few different hidden treasure ready to be explored. The Stockholm Archipelago in Sweden, with its hundreds of islands, offers a totally particular aggregate of nature and lifestyle. Visitors can sail thru the archipelago, preventing at picturesque islands with quaint villages, sandy beaches, and luxurious forests. The Åland Islands, placed amongst Sweden and Finland, also are famend for his or her natural splendor, providing scenic coastal landscapes, rocky seashores, and tranquil seashores.

In addition to its natural wonders, Scandinavia is likewise acknowledged for its determination to sustainable tourism. The place has implemented numerous initiatives to guard its pristine environments and decrease the effect of tourism on fragile ecosystems. From eco-motels and renewable electricity assets to accountable herbal world searching practices, Scandinavia is predominant the way in selling sustainable tour.

To in truth immerse oneself within the breathtaking landscapes of Scandinavia, it's far crucial to mission past the well-known factors of hobby and discover the lesser-appeared corners of this extremely good location. Whether it's far hiking through the untouched desolate tract of Swedish Lapland, sailing a number of the a ways flung islands of the Norwegian coast, or witnessing the unique plant life and fauna of Finnish countrywide parks, Scandinavia offers a wealth of opportunities to connect with nature and create unforgettable reminiscences.

In forestall, the landscapes of Scandinavia are not some thing short of high-quality. From the majestic fjords and towering mountains to the serene forests and enthralling archipelagos, this region is a paradise for nature fanatics and adventurers. The precise flowers and fauna, hidden gem stones, and herbal wonders add to the attraction of Scandinavia, inviting site visitors to embark on a journey of discovery and awe-inspiring beauty. So p.C. Your luggage, put on your trekking boots, and get prepared to be obsessed with the aid of the breathtaking landscapes of Scandinavia.

Chapter 12: Scandinavian Lifestyle

Overview of the Scandinavian way of lifestyles

Scandinavia, encompassing the global locations of Denmark, Norway, and Sweden, is known for its unique and incredible manner of lifestyles. The Scandinavian manner of lifestyles shows a mixture of cultural values, social guidelines, and ancient elements that have regular the place through the years. From their consciousness on equality and sustainability to their appreciation of nature and format, Scandinavians have fostered a manner of life that is each harmonious and cutting-edge.

One of the crucial aspect elements of the Scandinavian way of existence is the emphasis on egalitarianism. Scandinavian societies strive for equality in severa spheres, collectively with gender equality, earnings distribution, and social welfare. This is contemplated in pointers that assist regularly taking place healthcare, entire social safety structures, and sturdy tough work unions. The purpose is to create a society in which absolutely everyone has identical opportunities and get right of get entry to to to important offerings.

Furthermore, Scandinavians have a deep appreciation for nature and the out of doors. The area's cute landscapes, with massive forests, picturesque fjords, and pristine lakes, provide adequate possibilities for outdoor sports. It is not unusual to look people undertaking sports collectively with hiking, skiing, and biking. The connection with nature is not super seen as a supply of assignment however moreover as a way to preserve intellectual and physical properly-being.

Design is each different crucial part of the Scandinavian manner of existence. The area is renowned for its minimalist and realistic approach to layout, that is regularly characterised via clean traces, simplicity, and a focus on herbal substances. Scandinavian layout has recommended various fields, which include fixtures, structure, and fashion.

It combines aesthetics with capability, developing products and areas which may be visually appealing, practical, and robust.

Family and community play essential roles in the Scandinavian manner of lifestyles. The idea of "fika" in Sweden, for example, emphasizes the fee of taking regular breaks to revel in coffee and communique with pals, colleagues, or family people. This practice fosters social connections and a experience of network. Moreover, Scandinavians prioritize spending tremendous time with their families and often have bendy paintings schedules to cope with this.

Education is specially valued in Scandinavian societies. The training structures in Denmark, Norway, and Sweden are diagnosed for his or her emphasis on inclusivity, person development, and important thinking. Students are endorsed to discover their interests and pursue higher schooling. Education is generally free or heavily backed, making sure that everyone has identical get right of entry to to first-class education.

In phrases of healthcare, Scandinavian worldwide locations have superior green and comprehensive systems. Universal healthcare is furnished to all residents, regardless of their socioeconomic recognition. The healthcare systems cognizance on preventive care, early intervention, and affected character-focused strategies. This ensures that humans receive well timed and appropriate clinical remedy, foremost to better fitness effects.

Secrets to the famend Scandinavian paintings-lifestyles balance

The Scandinavian art work-life balance is often stylish and envied round the world. The region has controlled to strike a balance among artwork and private lifestyles, selling worker nicely-being and productivity. Several elements make a contribution to this particular artwork-life stability in Scandinavia.

One of the key elements is the implementation of bendy paintings preparations. Scandinavian worldwide places prioritize art work flexibility, allowing personnel to have manage over their walking hours and location. This promotes a more in shape art work-lifestyles integration, as human beings can higher manage their non-public commitments alongside their expert responsibilities. Flexible artwork preparations include options alongside aspect telecommuting, part-time work, and parental go away.

Another essential thing is the charge located on entertainment time. Scandinavians recognize the significance of relaxation and downtime for regular properly-being. They have shorter going for walks hours in assessment to many certainly one of a kind nations, and holidays are advocated and regularly legally mandated. Employers and co-people recognize and respect the need for people to recharge and spend time with family and pals. This emphasis on amusement time allows human beings to engage in hobbies, spend extremely good time with cherished ones, and prioritize self-care, which contributes to a greater healthy paintings-existence stability.

Moreover, Scandinavian international locations have sturdy social welfare systems that assist going for walks dad and mom. Generous parental go away recommendations are in location, allowing each mother and father to take day off paintings to attend to their youngsters. This promotes gender equality and encourages a more same distribution of childcare responsibilities. Childcare centers are also significantly available and of immoderate fine, allowing mother and father to transport back to art work with peace of thoughts.

Scandinavian places of work also foster a way of lifestyles of consider and autonomy. Employees are given a excessive diploma of duty and are trusted to control their paintings independently. Micromanagement is rare, and there can be a notion within the competence and professionalism of people. This autonomy effects in extended process satisfaction and a greater revel in of hard work-existence balance.

Another thing contributing to the Scandinavian artwork-existence balance is the prioritization of nicely-being and mental health. Mental fitness is taken drastically within the area, and measures are in region to beneficial aid employees' mental well-being. Companies offer get admission to to counseling services, stress manage applications, and sell open conversations about intellectual health. This emphasis on nicely-being creates a supportive paintings surroundings that values the overall fitness of employees.

Furthermore, the Scandinavian artwork way of life emphasizes efficiency and productivity for the duration of taking walks hours. With shorter strolling hours, personnel are encouraged to hobby on their duties, restriction distractions, and preserve a healthful artwork tempo. This inexperienced technique allows humans to finish their paintings in a well timed manner, lowering the want for extended hours and past everyday time.

Insight into hygge and precise cultural practices

Hygge, advised "hoo-ga," is a Danish time period that has won international interest in cutting-edge years. It encapsulates a unique cultural workout that emphasizes coziness, comfort, and a feel of nicely-being. Hygge isn't always most effective a phrase; it represents a manner of life this is deeply ingrained in Danish tradition. However, it is not the simplest cultural workout surely definitely really worth exploring in the Scandinavian region.

Hygge is all approximately growing a heat and alluring environment, whether it's far in a unmarried's home, at a occasion, or sincerely at some stage in non-public downtime. It involves embracing easy pleasures, which include taking component in a cup of heat tea, lighting candles, and surrounding oneself with easy blankets and cushty furniture. Hygge encourages mindfulness and being completely present in the 2nd, allowing humans to take delight inside the small joys of existence.

In addition to hygge, Scandinavian cultures produce other practices that make contributions to their not unusual well-being. For instance, "lagom" is a Swedish term that form of interprets to "virtually the proper quantity." It embodies the idea of stability and moderation in all factors of existence. Swedes attempt for a harmonious and sustainable life-style, fending off extra and valuing simplicity. Lagom encourages human beings to find contentment in having "sufficient" in area of continuously pursuing extra.

In Norway, there may be a exercising called "friluftsliv," which interprets to "open-air dwelling." Friluftsliv shows the Norwegian love for nature and outdoor activities. Norwegians actively looking for possibilities to connect to the herbal environment, whether it's trekking inside the mountains, fishing through the lakes, or snowboarding in the winter. This workout not handiest promotes physical nicely-being however additionally offers a sense of peace, tranqu ility, and a deep appreciation for the beauty of the herbal global.

Another cultural workout in Scandinavia is "fika." Originating from Sweden, fika refers back to the manner of existence of taking a harm, often with a cup of coffee or tea, and gambling a 2nd of rest with pals, circle of relatives, or colleagues. Fika is extra than best a coffee ruin; it's far a social ritual that promotes connection, communique, and a pause from the needs of regular existence. It is a time to unwind, proportion testimonies, and foster relationships.

Scandinavians actually have a strong experience of network and social harmony. This is apparent inside the concept of "dugnad" in Norway and "grannsamverkan" in Sweden. Dugnad refers back to the exercising of network volunteering, in which pals come together to work on shared obligations and responsibilities, consisting of cleaning public regions or organizing close by activities. Grannsamverkan, however, emphasizes community watch programs and network safety duties. These practices improve the bonds internal companies and create a sense of belonging and collective obligation.

Scandinavians furthermore price schooling and lifetime studying. The location has a strong tradition of imparting outstanding education from early teens via better schooling. Learning is visible as a lifelong pursuit, and possibilities for non-public and expert improvement are particularly valued. This willpower to schooling contributes to the general properly-being and intellectual increase of human beings in Scandinavian societies.

Furthermore, Scandinavian cultures prioritize sustainability and environmental recognition. There is a strong popularity of the effect humans have on this planet, and efforts are made to lessen carbon footprints and live in harmony with nature. Recycling, electricity performance, and sustainable layout practices are commonplace. This environmentally aware mind-set is deeply ingrained in the Scandinavian way of life.

Chapter 13: Scandinavian Folklore and Mythology

Scandinavian Folklore and Mythology

Scandinavian folklore and mythology are rich in charming recollections that have been passed down through generations. Rooted within the cultural traditions of the Nordic international locations, those tales provide a glimpse into the beliefs, values, and worldview of the human beings in the location. From legendary creatures to powerful gods, the folklore of Scandinavia is complete of marvel and appeal.

Scandinavian folklore includes a massive range of narratives, which includes myths, legends, and people testimonies. These tales have been often shared orally earlier than being written down, taking into consideration versions and variations over the years. They served as a manner to entertain, train, and provide an motive at the back of natural phenomena or historical events.

Tales of Legendary Creatures and Gods

One of the charming additives of Scandinavian folklore is the presence of mythical creatures. These beings, frequently portrayed as supernatural or mythical, executed sizable roles inside the memories and beliefs of the Nordic people.

1. The Norse Gods: At the coronary heart of Scandinavian mythology are the Norse gods, who ruled over the realms of Asgard, Midgard, and unique geographical regions. Odin, the chief god, modified into acknowledged for his records and knowledge. Thor, the god of thunder, wielded his powerful hammer Mjolnir to shield each gods and people. Loki, the trickster god, regularly induced mischief and have become a complicated character in the mythology.

2. Elves and Trolls: Scandinavian folklore is likewise full of tales of elves and trolls. Elves, known as "Alfar" in Old Norse, were regularly depicted as lovable, ethereal beings living in forests or hidden geographical regions. They were related to nature and every now and

then interacted with human beings. Trolls, however, had been often depicted as big, effective creatures that lived in caves or mountains. They have been diagnosed for their power and from time to time posed a chance to human beings.

3. Dragons and Serpents: Dragons and serpents additionally seem in Scandinavian folklore. The most well-known dragon in Norse mythology is Jormungandr, a big serpent that encircled the area and modified into destined to combat Thor in the course of Ragnarok, the cataclysmic struggle that marked the stop of the area. Dragons had been regularly portrayed as fearsome creatures guarding treasures or causing destruction.

Secrets Behind the Enduring Stories and Their Cultural Significance

The enduring reputation of Scandinavian folklore and mythology can be attributed to severa elements, collectively with their cultural significance and the undying subjects they explore. These memories keep to resonate with humans, supplying insights into the human revel in and presenting moral instructions.

1. Cultural Identity: Scandinavian folklore shows the cultural identity and data of the Nordic countries. The testimonies are intertwined with the landscapes, traditions, and records of the vicinity, serving as a source of countrywide delight and a way to preserve cultural history.

2. Moral Lessons: Many of the memories in Scandinavian folklore include moral training and values. They regularly find out difficulty topics of bravery, loyalty, honor, and the consequences of one's actions. The characters in those reminiscences characteristic role models or cautionary figures, education listeners and readers critical existence instructions.

three. Connection with Nature: Scandinavian folklore has a sturdy connection with nature. The natural landscape of the Nordic international places, with its mountains, forests, and fjords, is regularly depicted within the testimonies. Nature is personified, and legendary creatures are frequently associated with precise herbal elements, which encompass waterfalls, lakes, or the moon. These reminiscences fostered a deep reverence for the environment and an expertise of humanity's place within it.

four. Oral Tradition and Adaptation: The oral way of lifestyles done a important characteristic within the upkeep and transmission of Scandinavian folklore. The reminiscences have been exceeded down from technology to technology via oral storytelling, bearing in mind versions and variations to in shape the opportunities of different storytellers and their audiences. This dynamic nature of the folklore ensured its relevance and saved it alive at some point of the centuries.

5. Influence on Literature and Art: Scandinavian folklore has had a profound

have an effect on on literature and art work, each inside the Nordic international places and beyond. Many famend authors and artists have drawn concept from those memories, incorporating factors of Scandinavian mythology into their works. From J.R.R. Tolkien, who have become precipitated through Norse mythology whilst developing the arena of Middle-earth, to modern authors consisting of Neil Gaiman, the impact of Scandinavian folklore may be seen in severa varieties of inventive expression.

6. Contemporary Significance: Despite being rooted in historic instances, Scandinavian folklore continues to captivate and inspire human beings nowadays. Its situation topics of heroism, journey, and the struggle amongst suitable and evil resonate with mounted human stories. Moreover, the trendy surge in hobby in Nordic life-style, fueled through famous media along with television series and movies, has delivered Scandinavian folklore to a much broader global goal marketplace, similarly cementing its cultural importance.

Chapter 14: Scandinavian Festivals and Traditions

Overview of Traditional Scandinavian Festivals

Scandinavian countries are seemed for his or her rich cultural history and colourful traditions. Throughout the one year, numerous gala's and activities take area, showcasing the place's statistics, folklore, and customs. These celebrations supply human beings together, promoting network spirit and a experience of belonging. In this text, we're able to explore a top degree view of traditional Scandinavian festivals, delving into their importance and the sports activities that take place in the direction of those active events.

Midsummer Festival

One of the most critical festivals in Scandinavia is the Midsummer Festival, furthermore referred to as "Midsommar" in Sweden, "Juhannus" in Finland, and "Sankthansaften" in Norway. Celebrated sooner or later of the summer time solstice, generally on June 21st, this opposition marks the longest day of the one year and the advent of summer season.

During Midsummer, people gather in the geographical area or close to lakes and rivers to partake in numerous activities. Traditional customs include erecting a maypole, this is embellished with flowers and leaves. Dancing throughout the maypole is a commonplace practice, located with the useful useful resource of conventional parents music and songs.

Additionally, Midsummer festivities often encompass bonfires, in which people collect to socialize, sing, and revel in delicious meals. It is also a time while conventional video video games and competitions, in conjunction with tug-of-warfare and sack races, take area. The Midsummer Festival is a joyous occasion that lets in Scandinavians to embody nature, apprehend their cultural history, and feature fun the appearance of summer season.

St. Lucia's Day

St. Lucia's Day, additionally called "Luciadagen" in Sweden and "Luciadag" in Norway and Denmark, is a festival celebrated on December thirteenth. It honors St. Lucia, a third-century martyr who symbolizes slight and desire within the direction of the dark wintry climate months.

One of the large elements of St. Lucia's Day is the Lucia procession. A greater younger female is chosen to painting St. Lucia and wears a white robe with a red sash. She wears a crown of candles on her head, symbolizing the triumph of light over darkness. Accompanied with the aid of a procession of various kids, she visits houses, colleges, and hospitals, offering saffron buns and developing a music conventional songs.

St. Lucia's Day marks the beginning of the Christmas season in Scandinavia, and it's miles a time whilst human beings come together to spread warmth and cheer. The competition serves as a reminder of the significance of mild and want in some unspecified time in the future of the prolonged wintry weather nights.

Jokkmokk Winter Market

The Jokkmokk Winter Market is a completely precise opposition that takes vicinity inside the small metropolis of Jokkmokk, positioned in the northern a part of Sweden. This marketplace has been celebrated for over four hundred years and is considered one of the oldest ongoing marketplaces in the u . S ..

The opposition is held during the primary weekend of February and draws traffic from everywhere within the worldwide. It showcases the indigenous Sami way of lifestyles, imparting a glimpse into their conventional manner of lifestyles. At the market, you could find a widespread form of domestic made crafts, traditional Sami apparel, reindeer products, and nearby delicacies.

During the Jokkmokk Winter Market, cultural sports, stay shows, and exhibitions take area, supplying opportunities to find out about Sami traditions, track, and storytelling. Visitors can also participate in reindeer races and dog sledding competitions, immersing themselves in the wintry surroundings of the region.

Unique Customs and Traditions

Scandinavian festivals are acknowledged for their specific customs and traditions which have been surpassed down thru generations. These customs replicate the wealthy cultural records and close to connection to nature. Let's find out a number of the unique customs and traditions related to Scandinavian fairs.

Bonfires and Dancing

Bonfires play a sizable feature in lots of Scandinavian gala's, symbolizing the triumph of mild over darkness and averting evil spirits. During Midsummer, as cited in advance, bonfires are a not unusual characteristic of the celebrations. People collect across the bonfire, taking detail in its warm temperature and glow whilst creating a song and dancing collectively.

Traditional Attire

Traditional apparel holds a completely unique vicinity in Scandinavian fairs, representing the cultural history and satisfaction of the region. During festivals just like the Jokkmokk Winter Market, you could witness locals and visitors alike wearing conventional Sami garb. These vibrant and intricately designed clothes exhibit the craftsmanship and artistry of the Sami human beings.

In addition to the Sami clothing, fairs like St. Lucia's Day moreover function traditional costumes. The more younger female portraying St. Lucia wears a white robe with a red sash, symbolizing purity and martyrdom. This apparel, accompanied by way of manner of the enduring candle crown, creates a visually adorable and brilliant instance of the competition's hassle.

Food and Drink

Scandinavian gala's are an possibility to take delight in delicious conventional delicacies. Each competition has its non-public unique culinary delights, showcasing nearby flavors and elements.

During Midsummer, Scandinavians collect to revel in a festive meal called "smörgåsbord." This buffet-style night meal includes a whole lot of dishes consisting of pickled herring, meatballs, new potatoes, and fresh berries. It is a time to revel in the flavors of summer season and feature an excellent time the abundance of nature.

Similarly, the Jokkmokk Winter Market offers a threat to flavor traditional Sami dishes like "suovas" (smoked reindeer meat) and "gáhkku" (a sort of bread). These hearty and flavorsome delicacies provide a glimpse into the culinary traditions of the indigenous Sami culture.

Folklore and Mythology

Scandinavian festivals often include factors of folklore and mythology, including a touch of appeal to the celebrations. Stories and legends exceeded down via generations come to existence in a few unspecified time in the destiny of these events.

For instance, inside the path of Midsummer, it is believed that supernatural forces are at their maximum powerful. Folklore tells memories of hidden treasures, mythical creatures, and mischievous spirits. This mystical aspect affords an air of intrigue and pleasure to the festivities.

In a few areas, festivals additionally feature reenactments of historical mythical memories. These performances showcase the rich mythological ancient past of Scandinavia, captivating audiences and offering a deeper records of the cultural importance of these recollections.

Community and Togetherness

Perhaps the most tremendous subject matter throughout Scandinavian fairs is the revel in of community and togetherness they foster. These activities deliver people from all walks of existence together, developing a shared revel in that strengthens bonds and promotes a enjoy of belonging.

Whether it's miles dancing during the maypole in some unspecified time in the future of Midsummer, taking component within the Lucia procession, or exploring the Jokkmokk Winter Market, the fairs provide possibilities for locals and region site visitors alike to connect, proportion recollections, and create lasting recollections.

Unveiling the Secrets Behind Celebrated Scandinavian Events

Scandinavian festivals aren't quality wealthy in traditions however also steeped in records and cultural significance. They offer a window into the particular customs and practices that have formed the vicinity over the years. Let's delve deeper into a few celebrated

Scandinavian occasions and unveil the secrets and strategies and strategies within the lower lower back in their enduring popularity.

Sami National Day

On February sixth every three hundred and sixty five days, the Sami human beings, indigenous to the Arctic regions of Norway, Sweden, Finland, and Russia, have a laugh their National Day. This day marks the repute quo of the Sami Parliament, which targets to sell and protect Sami rights, language, and life-style.

The Sami National Day is an event for the Sami human beings to reveal off their colourful historical past thru severa cultural sports. Traditional reindeer races, yoik creating a song (a form of conventional Sami tune), and colourful parades are a number of the highlights of the celebrations. The event presents an possibility to find out about the Sami manner of lifestyles, their reindeer herding traditions, and their deep connection to the Arctic environment.

Crayfish Party

The Crayfish Party, called "Kräftskiva" in Swedish, is a cherished summer season lifestyle in Sweden. This completely happy celebration takes region in August, usually in out of doors settings, wherein buddies and circle of relatives acquire to bask in an abundance of crayfish, determined with the aid of manner of making a music, laughter, and merriment.

The manner of existence of the Crayfish Party dates once more to the 19th century on the same time as crayfish harvesting changed into strictly regulated. After policies had been lifted, the Swedes embraced this opportunity to have fun with gusto. Decorated with lanterns and embellished with paper hats, participants engage in active conversation, sing conventional eating songs, and interact in extremely good consuming video video games.

The Crayfish Party represents a joyous celebration of summer season, friendship, and the bounties of the sea. It's a time whilst Swedes come collectively to satisfaction in the delectable flavors of crayfish, located through some of trouble dishes like Västerbotten cheese pie and crispbread.

Christmas Markets

Christmas markets hold a special vicinity in Scandinavian way of life and are eagerly awaited every year. These festive markets, known as "Julmarknad" in Swedish, are held within the course of the Advent season in numerous towns and towns across Scandinavia.

The markets are decorated with twinkling lighting fixtures, festive decorations, and the attractive aromas of mulled wine, gingerbread, and roasted almonds. Stalls offer diverse hand made presents, adorns, and traditional treats. Visitors can browse through the stalls, savoring the Christmas spirit and locating particular treasures.

One of the most renowned Christmas markets is the Tivoli Gardens Christmas Market in Copenhagen, Denmark. This captivating marketplace features leisure park rides, ice-skating, and a captivating moderate show, growing a mystical surroundings for web site site visitors of each age.

The Battle of Halden

The Battle of Halden, additionally referred to as "Trefningene ved Halden," is a ancient reenactment event that takes vicinity in Halden, Norway. The warfare commemorates the sports of the Swedish-Norwegian War of 1814 and the subsequent signing of the Convention of Moss, which paved the manner for Norway's independence from Sweden.

Printed in the USA
CPSIA information can be obtained
at www.ICGtesting.com
LVHW022337291123
765332LV00041B/1417